Overcoming Common Problems Series

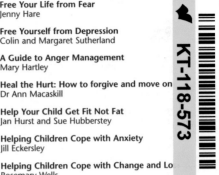

Overcoming Common Problems Series

Coping with Headaches and Migraine

Alison Frith MSc BSc (Hons) RGN MICR has run clinical research trials in migraine and headaches at the City of London Migraine Clinic since 1999. Alison trained in nursing at the Middlesex Hospital, London and then read Human Sciences at University College, London. She combines her nursing and science background to work with people daily as they cope with their headaches. Alison has migraine herself, which gives her a special perspective. She is co-editor of *ABC of Headache*, and has co-authored papers in scientific journals. Alison was awarded the accolade of 'Best Healthcare Professional 2008' at the Migraine Heroes Healthcare Awards, run by Migraine Action, a national charity for people with migraine and other headaches.

Overcoming Common Problems Series

Selected titles

A full list of titles is available from Sheldon Press,
36 Causton Street, London SW1P 4ST, and on our website at
www.sheldonpress.co.uk

Overcoming Common Problems

Coping with Headaches and Migraine

ALISON FRITH

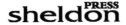

First published in Great Britain in 2009
Sheldon Press
36 Causton Street
London SW1P 4ST

The author and publisher have made every effort to ensure that the
external website and email addresses included in this book are correct and
up to date at the time of going to press. The author and publisher are not
responsible for the content, quality or continuing accessibility of the sites.

British Library Cataloguing-in-Publication Data
A catalogue record for this book is available from the British Library

ISBN 978-1-84709-038-6

1 3 5 7 9 10 8 6 4 2

Typeset by Fakenham Photosetting Ltd, Fakenham, Norfolk
Printed in Great Britain by Ashford Colour Press

Produced on paper from sustainable forests

In loving memory of my father Ron.

Contents

Acknowledgements

Firstly, many thanks to all those who have attended the City of London Migraine Clinic, talked to me about their headaches and offered themselves so willingly to participate in our clinical studies. Your contributions help us to discover new ways of coping and offer hope to others.

Thank you to Dr Anne MacGregor, Clinical Research Director at the City of London Migraine Clinic. Working with you is as joyful as it is challenging. Thank you for being a mentor, for gently encouraging me to achieve new things and for being a special friend.

All my wonderful colleagues at the City of London Migraine Clinic are also greatly appreciated. I have never been happier in my work, and I know that is good for my migraine. Drs Nat Blau and Marcia Wilkinson, who set up the Clinic as a charity almost 30 years ago, created a very special place. I am very proud to work with you to help people cope with their headaches.

I also thank my husband Alan, whose sense of humour always brightens my day. Thank you for keeping me fed and hydrated – I don't always practise what I preach, and you have kept away many a migraine.

Also deserving thanks are my mother Cathy, brother Andrew, sister Catherine and my many friends for unfailing support.

Finally, thank you to Fiona Marshall at Sheldon Press. I am grateful for your encouragement, patience and wise words.

Alison Frith

Foreword

Although most headaches and migraines are not life-threatening, the profound effect they can have on your ability to function and carry out your usual daily activities means that they are now recognized by the World Health Organization as one of the leading causes of disability. But it has been a battle to gain this attention – for centuries headaches have been ignored, or worse they have been seen solely as a psychological problem. Fortunately, recent research confirms that headaches have an organic basis and there are now specific and effective drugs to help prevent and treat the most severe types of headaches, particularly migraine and cluster headache.

However, drugs are only a part of managing headaches; an understanding of what the condition is caused by and how treatments work can make the difference between being in control of migraine and feeling controlled by it. It is not just you who can benefit from this understanding – family, friends and employers are also indirectly affected by migraine.

Alison Frith is well placed to share her expertise in helping you cope with your headaches and migraines. It has been a privilege to work with her over the past nine years. She has the advantage of writing from the heart, having experienced her own battle with migraine. But she also has the rare ability of being able to look objectively at the problems, learning from the good and the bad experiences of the patients that she sees every day.

I have no doubt that you will find this book an invaluable source of information to help you understand and gain better control of your headaches.

Dr Anne MacGregor
The City of London Migraine Clinic

Abbreviations

CBT = cognitive behavioural therapy
CHC = combined hormonal contraceptive
CSD = cortical spreading depression
GP = general practitioner
HOOF = Home Oxygen Order Form
HRT = hormone replacement therapy
5-HT = 5-hydroxytriptamine
5-HTP = 5-hydroxytryptophan
mg = milligrams
MOH = medication over-use headache
NSAID = non-steroidal anti-inflammatory drug
OUCH = Organization for the Understanding of Cluster Headache
PFO = patent foramen ovale
PMS = premenstrual syndrome
TENS = transcutaneous electrical nerve stimulation
TTH = tension-type headache

Introduction

A personal experience

Matron escorted me back to the nurses' home just after midnight. Despite her obvious concern and my dazed state, I could tell she was really cross. I was a nurse on night duty in charge of 28 patients and now I would have to be replaced, leaving another ward short staffed. And just because I had a headache.

I was in no fit state to care for my patients that night. On matron's ward round I got everyone muddled up and couldn't get my words out. I excused myself to be violently sick in the sluice room, where the smell of disinfectant seemed noxious and bored into my brain. When I staggered back my hat was lop-sided and my own vomit was splattered down my starched apron and over my shoes. Matron knew that there was something very wrong. My head was splitting in half with the pain as if someone had stabbed it. I looked at the crisp, white linen on an empty bed and longed to lie down, completely still and surrounded by darkness. Just long enough for the pain to ease, and the pounding to stop. Quietness for a few moments. Perhaps then I could carry on ...

Back in my room I was so sick in the basin that my stomach hurt as well as my head. I found some relief sitting on the floor with my temple pressed hard against the cold, porcelain bowl. I cried with the pain and with the guilt too. I felt I had let down my colleagues and all my patients who needed me. When I finally stood up and saw my sunken eyes reflected in the mirror, I was truly horrified at how grey and ill I looked. Some of those in my care had looked healthier than me!

I slept all that night and all next day. When I reported for duty that evening the pain had gone, but I felt that my head was filled with cotton wool. I struggled with my work. It was several days until I felt well again. I tried to put the headache out of my mind. But then it happened again.

How I coped with my headaches

What I know now, but didn't know then, was that I was having severe migraine attacks. I didn't realize that you needn't have bright lights in your eyes for it to be migraine. My headaches had become much worse and I thought they might be killing me. Like many nurses in training I had often mistakenly diagnosed myself with brain tumours and other nasty illnesses. It was time for me to get help, and I went to my doctor.

For me, the important first step in coping was getting help when I needed it and identifying the headache, which came as a relief. The next steps were to learn about my migraine, discover my own triggers and make changes to aspects of my lifestyle that were not helping me at all. As a young nurse I was always anxious, making sure that I was doing my best, and the wards could be hot, stressful places for both staff and patients. Irregular hours were another problem outside my control. I would barely recover from one week of night duty before it was my turn again.

I had to make changes. I discovered that infrequent meals and lack of fluids were significant personal triggers that I could do something about. I forced myself to drink more water even when I wasn't thirsty and had regular snacks. I also stayed awake on my first day off night duty, so that I could recover my sleeping pattern more quickly. These simple strategies made a real difference to the frequency of my attacks.

Learning to cope with my migraine has been a journey that has taken many years. It is a happy coincidence that I am now working at the City of London Migraine Clinic. It is a subject very close to my heart. I only wish I knew back then what I know now. I could have understood earlier that migraine is more than just headache and is really a whole process. Our doctors and patients often describe migraine as kind of body 'power cut'. No wonder I would always feel ghastly for days!

My migraine attacks still happen from time to time, despite my best efforts. So, importantly, I've had to find treatments that work for me. These have changed a few times, and working at the Clinic has helped me know what to do for the best. Keeping one step ahead is ongoing. You can't forget that you are prone to migraine attacks – they don't let you. However, by understanding my own migraine and triggers and by finding effective treatments, I have gained more control. I have eventually learned to cope with my attacks. Although they occasionally stop me in my tracks, I usually know why. I no longer live in fear of migraine, as I have done at times in my life.

Coping with headaches

Although there are no miracle cures for migraine or other kinds of headache, there are effective treatments and so much you can do to help yourself. A combination of approaches can really make a difference.

I believe that it is important to try to recognize what type of headaches you have. This can be difficult because even experts argue over names, and more than one headache type can occur at the same time. However, the reassurance of knowing what you are dealing with will stop you from worrying about it. You can then concentrate on how best to deal with the headaches. These are the first steps to assuming control and learning to cope. Unfortunately, there are no quick fixes. It isn't easy – often it is a process of trial and error, and sometimes there can be relapses. You will still have to make allowances for your headaches, but aim never to allow them to control you, because you control them. I know this because it is what I am doing myself.

The global burden of headaches

People who have troublesome headaches understand the major impact they can have on family life, social life and employment. Not only do they stop you from doing what you want, but even when you haven't got a headache, you can be living in dread of the next one. They can also be very disabling and blight the lives of you *and* your family.

We are not alone with our headaches. Estimates suggest that up to ten million people in the UK regularly have migraine and other headaches. Headaches account for about 20 per cent of days off sick from work. The cost to the UK economy could be more than £1.5 billion per year, because on any single day 100,000 people are absent because of a migraine attack. Additionally, we all know that even if you do go to work with a headache you will not be very productive.

This isn't confined to the UK. The initiative 'Lifting the Burden, the Global Campaign to Reduce the Burden of Headache Worldwide' (see Useful addresses at the end of this book) recognizes all headaches as a global issue. Reflecting this, migraine is ranked by the World Health Organization as being in the world's top 20 most disabling diseases. For women it is ranked number 12. If other types of headache were included, the ranking could be even higher!

If more people were helped to manage their headaches, they would miss less time from work and home life, lessening the burden for both individuals and society. However, despite being the most common neurological disorder, headache is not a priority. Doctors and people who don't have disabling headaches (or know someone who does) often regard headaches as trivial. Perhaps this is because nearly everyone gets a mild headache from time to time and thinks nothing of it. Perhaps it is also because common headaches are intermittent and not usually life-threatening or catching. As a result, migraine and headaches are often not properly diagnosed or treated, specialist headache services are not widely available and research funding is inadequate.

Your own headache burden

People with headaches do not help the situation. Because of the stigma of having 'just a headache', many of us try to ignore headaches, pretend we don't have them or simply rely on too many over-the-counter medications that don't work. Sometimes we spend money on treatments, hoping for cures that just don't exist. Also, like me, many people fail to recognize that they could have migraine, or simply don't visit their doctors to find out. Because medical treatments are available for most kinds of common headache, I encourage you to seek help if you need it and to keep looking until you find it. There might not be cures, but most people can find relief. By combining effective medical treatments with healthy living, complementary therapies that work for you and a positive approach, you really can lessen your burden.

How this book can help you cope with your headaches

I understand about trying to cope with headaches because of my own experience, but I am also privileged to work with leading headache doctors. Drs Nat Blau and Anne MacGregor, Medical Directors at the City of London Migraine Clinic, and their dedicated team of doctors work tirelessly every day to help people who have headaches. We listen to patients' problems and help them to find coping solutions through care, effective treatments and new research.

In this book I would like to share with you some simple ideas that may help you to cope better with your headaches. I have learned these over the years through my own experience and from talking to people with headaches about what works for them. These are the kinds of things that I would have liked to have known when I first discovered that I had migraine. It isn't just about going to the doctor and taking tablets – far from it. It is more about listening to your body and what it might be trying to tell you when you get a headache.

Throughout the book I have indicated where there is scientific evidence for ideas and treatments and where there is not. Surprisingly little robust evidence is available. For those of us battling with our headaches, it isn't about research (although do consider taking part in a study if you can). Instead, it is about finding what helps you best to live your life with as few headaches as possible and without living in dread of them. When a headache does come, as it will from time to time, you need to be able to deal with it effectively.

This book aims to help you cope better in the following ways.

- Helping you to recognize your headaches. What kind of headaches do you have? Could they be serious and when should you see your doctor?
- Helping you to understand more about your headaches. This includes what they are, who gets them and the likelihood of improvement.
- Showing you how to cope with and without drugs. You need to find a strategy that works for you. Combining strategies may help you to cope better.
- Providing specific advice for headaches in women. By virtue of hormones, women have more headaches and migraine than men at different stages in their lives.
- Showing you how to help yourself. Looking after your health and your diet and being willing to help yourself can make a real difference to coping.
- Helping you know what to expect from medical help. By being prepared you can get the best out of medical help, because sometimes you can't cope by yourself.

I hope you will find useful ideas to help you to cope with your headaches. Sometimes the smallest changes can make the biggest difference. I know lack of fluids is a strong trigger for my migraine. As I tell our research trialists, new drugs aren't everything – I must drink the water on my desk and not just look at it.

1

Recognizing your headache: is it serious?

Headaches are so common that only about two per cent of people claim never to have had one. For the majority, headaches occur once in a while and are not too troublesome. They could be due to tension, a cold or flu, or just over-indulgence in alcohol – a hangover headache. One or two painkillers are enough to ease them.

These headaches are manageable and, apart from occasional inconvenience, they don't worry us too much. But what if your headaches are a sign of something serious? Having a stroke or a brain tumour is what people worry about most, especially if headaches are severe or frequent.

Fortunately, brain tumours are rare. More importantly, fewer than ten per cent of brain tumours present with just a headache. A serious underlying cause represents less than one per cent of people who go to their doctor with headache. This is all reassuring, but it is important to know when you *should* see your doctor.

When you should see your doctor

Sometimes a doctor's reassurance is as helpful as any therapy you might try, so see your doctor if you are worried about your headache for any reason.

Headaches on their own without any other symptoms are rarely a cause for concern. The following headaches and symptoms are prompts to seek medical advice. They do not necessarily mean that you have serious headaches, just that you should seek a proper diagnosis.

- Headaches beginning after the age of 50.
- A new headache in a child under the age of 12.
- Sudden onset of a new or 'worst ever' headache, especially if very severe, abrupt or explosive, which peaks within minutes. 'Thunderclap headache' is a fitting description.
- Worsening of headache and/or associated symptoms over days or weeks.

- Physical problems that are not typically associated with headaches or continuing in the absence of headache. These include changes or loss of consciousness, fits, severe confusion, blindness, weakness of limbs, loss of sensation, and pains in the face, jaw or mouth.
- Headache with a fever not caused by something obvious like having a cold or flu.
- Headache with prolonged nausea and vomiting.
- Headache brought on by exertion, including coughing, sneezing, stooping, exercise or straining on the toilet.
- Headache associated with sexual activity, before or during orgasm.
- New or unusual symptoms or a change in pattern in your longstanding headaches, such as greater frequency, intensity or duration.
- A new headache if you do not normally have headaches.
- Onset of headache if you have had cancer, HIV/AIDS or immune deficiency.
- Onset of headache if you have had a head injury.
- Headache at the same time as high blood pressure.
- Headache with an aura lasting for longer than one hour or associated with weakness of your arms or legs (see Chapter 2).
- An aura without a headache if you haven't previously been diagnosed with migraine with aura.
- An aura for the first time if you are using a combined oral contraceptive.
- Psychological changes associated with headaches, such as marked changes in behaviour or personality, or failure to cope at work or school.

Different kinds of headaches

Doctors group headaches for the purposes of diagnosis, treatment and research.

Primary headaches

A primary headache (and associated symptoms) is the term used when the headache is the disease itself, as opposed to a headache that is caused by (or secondary to) another illness, infection or injury. Sometimes described as benign headaches, primary headaches on their own are not life-threatening, although they have all been described as 'quality of life-threatening'. They include migraine, tension-type headache (TTH) and cluster headache.

Secondary headaches

These headaches are caused by another process, injury or disease of the head and neck, including blood vessels, bones, sinuses, eyes, ears, nose, teeth, mouth and face. They include stroke, brain tumour or infection (e.g. meningitis). Substances such as drugs and alcohol, or withdrawal from them, are also causes.

Secondary headaches are excluded by a doctor before a diagnosis of a primary headache is made. They are outside the scope of this book because they need specific medical treatments, rather than self-help measures.

Recognizing headaches

Migraine

Migraine is a common, primary headache. It is not always recognized. The main feature is a severe 'sick' headache that lasts from a few hours to several days. You are usually well between attacks, which are episodic weekly or years apart. If your headache occurs every day, then you may be having migraine and another headache. Treatments you are taking may be causing more frequent headaches. (See Chapters 10, 11 and 12.)

People wonder whether there is a difference between a headache and a migraine. A migraine attack is much more than just a headache, which is only one of the symptoms. If you are not sure whether you have migraine, answer the I-D Migraine Test™ questions. There is more information about recognizing and coping with migraine in Chapters 2–5.

The I-D Migraine Test™

During the past 3 months, did you have any of the following symptoms together with a headache?
- You felt nauseous/sick?
- Light bothered you (a lot more than when you didn't have a headache)?
- Your headache limited your ability to work, study, play or do what you wanted to for at least one day?

If you answered 'yes' to at least two out of three questions, then it is likely that the headache was migraine. (Reference: Lipton and colleagues, 2003.)

Tension-type headache

More common than migraine, TTH is the 'normal' kind of headache that happens from time to time, caused by muscular tension or stress. Sometimes described as a tight band or squeezing around the head, there are no distinguishing symptoms and you don't usually feel sick. If you need to treat TTH, one or two painkillers are normally effective. It can become troublesome if it starts to happen more often or if painkillers lose their ability to control the pain. You can read more about TTH in Chapters 6 and 7. Also look at Chapters 10, 11 and 12 if your headaches are happening on most days.

Cluster headache

Unlike migraine and TTH, cluster headache is a rare primary headache. It is not widely recognized, properly diagnosed or treated, but in its typical form it can be identifiable. Some people visiting the City of London Migraine Clinic have told us that they recognized their headache from information on our website. Another sent a colleague to us because he recognized symptoms that were identical to his own!

Not to be confused with migraine, which can 'cluster' together in days of severe attacks, cluster headache is different. It has several distinguishing features. The headache is excruciating and is described as 'suicide headache'. Short attacks of pain lasting minutes to hours occur in bouts of one to eight per day. These bouts can persist for six to twelve weeks, and can happen once or twice in a year. During attacks you may be very restless or agitated. On the affected side you may notice eye changes and a blocked or running nostril. The other side is totally unaffected.

If you think you have cluster headache, then you need medical advice because self-help measures don't work. There are effective treatments and you can read more in Chapters 8 and 9.

2

Migraine: causes and triggers

Christine, 27
'People think that migraine is just a bad headache. That is only part of it! I'm sick for hours on end, can't do anything except lie down and feel awful. It takes me days to recover properly and I lose time out of my life. I'm getting married next year and already I'm worrying about whether I'll get a migraine on my wedding day ...'

Tackling migraine requires a dual approach – prevention and treatment. Unfortunately, like me, many people don't even realize that they have it! They miss out on effective management strategies and fail to cope. Additionally, having other types of headaches at the same time can confuse matters. Try the I-D Migraine Test™ in Chapter 1 to find out whether you are a 'migraineur'. Recognizing your migraine and understanding how it affects you can allow you to cope better. Everyone is different and migraines vary between attacks in the same person.

What is migraine?

Migraine is a primary headache, like TTH and cluster headache, and it may co-exist with them. There are no specific tests to identify migraine. It is diagnosed by a doctor based on your headache description and symptoms.

The word migraine derives from 'hemicrania', meaning headache on one side. The one-sided head pain is typically severe and pulsating. You can feel or be sick and become sensitive to sound, light and smell. One of the features of migraine is that it is a disabling type of headache. If migraine doesn't stop you from doing what you were doing, it really slows you down – a 'power cut' process.

The migraine may or may not be accompanied by an aura, usually involving distinctive visual disturbances – this is different from the blurred vision that often accompanies a migraine headache. Most migraineurs do not in fact have aura.

Migraine is a recurring disorder. It occurs on average every four to six weeks. Some people have migraine infrequently, with gaps of a year or more at a time. Others can have it much more frequently, with barely a week's respite during a bad run. Migraine lasts from four hours to three days. If the migraine goes away and returns less than two days later, it is part of the same migraine. This whole period is called a 'migraine attack'. Typically, people recover and are completely well in between attacks.

Phases of a migraine attack

In a migraine attack, the headache itself is only one of five phases. These are the warning phase, the aura, the headache, the resolution and the recovery. Understanding the phases will help you to cope with what is happening. During an attack, though, it is not always obvious which phase of the attack you are in.

Phase 1: warning symptoms of a migraine attack

This prodromal or premonitory phase is common, affecting two-thirds of migraineurs. You may notice a few aches, especially around your neck, and may not feel quite yourself. Warning symptoms can be one extreme or the other:

- mood – feeling very happy or miserable or irritable;
- behaviour – over-active or lethargic and clumsy;
- appetite – not feeling hungry, feeling sick or craving certain foods, often chocolate;
- bowels – either constipation or diarrhoea; and
- fluid balance – feeling thirsty, wanting to pass more urine or water retention.

Neurological symptoms of migraine can begin as:

- yawning – sometimes more than usual, as if you cannot stop;
- inability to find your words;
- inability to focus your eyes or blurred vision (*not* migraine aura, which is a distinctive set of symptoms – see 'Phase 2', below);
- sensitivity to light, sound and smells; and
- feeling very tired and unable to concentrate.

These changes can be very subtle and develop for up to 24 hours before the headache even starts. You may not be able to recognize them at the time, but your family and friends might. More than once a doctor at the City of London Migraine Clinic has asked me whether I have a migraine. I've denied this, only for it develop some hours later! They notice me looking paler, yawning, muddling up my words or being rather crabby. It's often a day when I've missed my lunch, with no chance to slow down and eat and drink something. These are not symptoms I can always take notice of, but if you can avoid some of your triggers then you may be able to stop an attack developing.

Phase 2: migraine aura

A typical migraine aura is a distinctive set of visual, sensory and speech symptoms. You may have one or all of these neurological features, together or in succession.

- *Visual aura symptoms* account for 99 per cent of migraine auras. They take the form of blind spots, distorted vision like looking through a broken mirror, flashing lights, zigzags (fortification spectra) or an expanding shimmering dot with a jagged edge, like a crescent (scintillating scotoma). You may have a sensation of a visual disturbance marching across your field of vision, from one side to the other. It may appear to affect only one eye, but if you cover it you will find that the other eye is affected too. This is because 'visual' aura symptoms are from your brain. They have been reported in a woman with migraine who was born without eyes.
- *Sensory aura symptoms* account for a third of auras, usually occurring with visual symptoms. Typically, pins and needles, tingling or numbness starts in your fingers and moves up your arm to your face and tongue. The legs are not usually affected. The sensation is one-sided and is not normally associated with weakness or loss of power.
- *Speech disturbances associated with aura* cause temporary difficulty finding your words (dysphasia). This occurs less often and is usually in association with visual and/or sensory symptoms.

The aura symptoms are part of the migraine attack but start and stop *before* the migraine headache begins. You return to normal when they are gone. Onset is not sudden but gradual, over at least five minutes. They can last up to an hour in total, with an average of 20 minutes. The headache usually begins up to an hour or so later.

Although auras vary between attacks, most migraineurs become used to their typical symptoms. If you get an aura for the first time, if it lasts longer than usual or if symptoms do not return to normal, then consult your doctor. Persistent loss of strength in an arm or leg is not a typical aura, although it can occur in hemiplegic migraine.

Phase 3: migraine headache and associated symptoms

The headache is the same regardless of whether it was preceded by an aura. It usually pulsates or pounds. It can be around the temple or anywhere on one side of the head. Unlike TTH, it is moderate or severe, not usually mild. Your neck can also be painful during a migraine and the build up of an attack.

Sometimes the headache isn't the worst symptom, as your whole body seems to shut down. Accompanying symptoms are nausea, and you can be very sick. You are also sensitive to sound, light and smell. They don't have to be particularly loud, bright or bad, but during a migraine they can seem intolerable. You seem overly sensitive to everything, and things that wouldn't normally hurt like brushing your hair can be painful. Feelings of depression during a migraine can be overwhelming. This is more than just being miserable because you have a headache, and may be related to brain chemicals involved in migraine attacks.

Routine activity and movement aggravate migraine; you just want to lie down in a dark room. You look pale, have no energy, can't eat, concentrate or do anything properly, and generally feel rotten.

Phase 4: resolution of the migraine attack

The way that a migraine attack resolves varies between people and between attacks in individuals. We don't know much about how or why attacks switch off.

Some people sleep it off, feeling much better when they wake. Others, unfortunately, wake up and the migraine is still there. Some migraineurs, particularly children, find that once they have been sick (sometimes violently) they have a sense of relief, as though the pressure of the pain has gone. Other people need to take medication and some just let the attack run its course.

Phase 5: recovery from the migraine attack

This postdromal phase describes how you feel after the attack and can vary. Many migraineurs feel completely washed out and drained for at least another day afterward. They can feel quite low and lethargic. Others, though, can feel high – almost euphoric even – and they rush about, probably making up for lost time!

Types of migraine

There are three main types of migraine.

Migraine without aura

Previously known as 'common migraine', this affects about 70 per cent of migraineurs. Some women experience this around their period ('menstrual migraine'; see Chapter 13).

Migraine with aura

You don't have to experience aura to have a migraine attack. Previously known as 'classical migraine', this only affects about 30 per cent of migraineurs.

About 20 per cent of people with migraine experience both types of migraine attacks – that is, some with aura and some without. Only around 10 per cent of people have attacks exclusively with aura.

Michael, 46

'I have had migraine since my early twenties. It always starts in my left eye with a bright spot of light, which gradually gets bigger and brighter. I can't see properly. I close my eyes and it is still there. Sometimes I get a prickly feeling in my fingers that spreads up my arm too. I now know it is the start of a migraine attack, and a headache will soon follow.'

Migraine aura without headache

This represents about one per cent of migraine attacks. It is more common in older people and those who have had migraine with aura in the past.

Rare types of migraine

If you suspect that you have any of the following rare types of migraine, see your doctor. You may need to see a specialist too.

Basilar-type migraine

This is migraine with aura with additional symptoms before the headache. Symptoms arise from the brain stem. They include slurred speech, ringing in the ears, severe dizziness, temporary vision loss and occasionally loss of consciousness. Although triptans are not usually recommended for this type of migraine, other standard treatments can be prescribed.

Hemiplegic migraine

This is migraine with aura with weakness or paralysis of the arm and leg on one side of the body. The weakness or paralysis can precede migraine headache, or can continue for the duration of the attack. Your doctor must diagnose this type of migraine, because symptoms are similar to those of stroke. It can run in families, in which case it is called 'familial hemiplegic migraine'.

Retinal migraine

Temporary blindness, blind spots or bright lights in one eye only may be retinal migraine. Migraine headache may begin during the symptoms or for up to one hour afterward. Eye examination is normal, and your doctor will exclude visual disturbances caused by other factors.

Status migrainosus

This is when migraine lasts for longer than the usual 72 hours. It may last for several weeks. Occasionally, hospitalization is required if dehydration occurs because of persistent vomiting. Triptans (anti-migraine medications) are usually very effective at treating migraine, but sometimes the symptoms repeatedly return on consecutive days, resulting in ongoing symptoms.

Who gets migraine?

Migraine is common, affecting about 10–12 per cent of the population. In the UK, estimates suggest that six million people are affected and that 190,000 migraine attacks occur every day.

Migraine typically first occurs during the teenage years or early twenties and usually before the age of 40. It can occur in children, with boys and girls equally affected until puberty. Over a life time about 25 per cent of women have migraine, as compared with eight per cent of men. Migraine is usually worse for women in their thirties and forties, whereas for men it remains more constant over the life time.

In the Europe and the USA, migraine is more common in Caucasian people than in other races. We don't yet understand the genes involved in migraine. Specific genes have been identified for the rare familial hemiplegic migraine, but we don't know how relevant this is to typical migraine with and without aura. Migraine does seem to run in families, with people inheriting a tendency to have migraine. Environmental factors may then trigger migraine attacks in people who are susceptible.

Causes of migraine attacks

The exact causes of migraine are still unknown and are the focus of considerable research and debate. We are not sure how attacks are switched on, maintained or switched off.

What causes the start of a migraine attack?

Migraine is now thought to be a disorder that primarily originates from neurological changes in brain chemistry. Blood vessels in the brain then constrict and swell, causing headache.

Current theories suggest that those of us with migraine have over-excitable brains, even when we don't actually have a migraine. An inherited low threshold makes us sensitive to migraine triggers, which act as stimuli to provoke migraine attacks in us but not in those without migraine. Changes in various chemicals within the brain, including calcium, magnesium and glutamate, have been implicated in the excitation process in migraine. This is when nerve cells (neurones) become over-active and we get a migraine attack.

The neurones transmit pain signals by sending electrical and chemical messages. One of many chemical messengers (neurotransmitters) implicated in migraine is serotonin (also known as 5-Hydroxytriptamine, or 5-HT). Serotonin could be important at the start of an attack, when levels are initially high and then drop. Before a headache even starts, changing serotonin levels may change blood vessels and increase blood clotting as platelets in the blood clump together. Brain function in certain areas of the brain, particularly the brain stem and hypothalamus, becomes disrupted. As the hypothalamus controls appetite, thirst, sleep and mood, this could account for the warning symptoms before a migraine attack. Research is currently being conducted on parts of the brain stem to see how they might generate a migraine attack.

What causes a migraine aura?

A neurological process called 'cortical spreading depression' (CSD) has been proposed to account for migraine aura. We don't know whether CSD is important in initiating migraine, exactly how it starts and whether it is significant in those who don't have migraine aura.

The process is believed to begin when a stimulus provokes excitation of nerves to become more electrically active. A wave of decreased electrical nerve activity then spreads across a part of the brain called the cortex. This has many functions, including controlling your vision and senses. CSD could account for the various symptoms experienced during an aura at the start of an attack. CSD may be associated with blood vessel constriction and reduced blood flow in the cortex. It has been suggested that all of these changes are linked to aura, because the rate of CSD moving across the cortex is similar to visual symptoms moving across your visual field before a migraine attack.

What causes the migraine headache?

Many complex processes in the nervous system are likely to play a role. Release of serotonin initially causes blood vessels in the outer layer of the brain (meninges) to constrict and later they swell as serotonin levels drop. Serotonin binds to special receptors throughout the brain, including on the trigeminal nerve. Branches of this sensory nerve spread from the outer meninges to deep within the brain stem. They are responsible for the transmission of pain sensation that is relayed to the sensory areas of the cortex.

When the blood vessels swell, they irritate the surrounding nerves of the trigeminal system. Various inflammatory substances are released, including calcitonin gene-related peptide. This causes more swelling of blood vessels and further activation of the nerves. These changes in blood vessels, blood flow and nerve sensitization could account for the pulsating pain of the headache, nausea and other migraine symptoms.

What causes a migraine attack to end?

The attack ends when pain and inflammatory processes subside, which can take several days. Painkillers and anti-inflammatory drugs can help to stop migraine attacks. Sometimes, anti-migraine medications that target the migraine process specifically are more effective.

Direct injection of serotonin has too many blood vessel constricting side effects, but triptans are highly effective once a migraine headache begins. These serotonin receptor agonist drugs activate receptors and mimic the effect of serotonin. They are believed to switch off an attack by preventing swelling of the blood vessels and, importantly, by stopping release of inflammatory substances. Drugs that block serotonin receptors (e.g. methysergide) and drugs that influence serotonin levels (e.g. anti-epileptic drugs) can be effective as migraine preventatives. There is currently research into developing new medications that block the action of substances such as calcitonin gene-related peptide and glutamate. These could be important in preventing and treating migraine attacks in the future.

Common triggers for migraine

A recent study showed that 76 per cent of migraineurs can identify triggering factors for attacks. It usually takes more than a single trigger. Here are some common triggers.

- Diet – missing meals, delayed meals, hunger and caffeine withdrawal.
- Dehydration – not drinking enough water.
- Alcohol – migraineurs are more susceptible to the effects of alcohol.
- Sleep – too little or too much can trigger migraine. Migraine typically occurs at the weekend when sleep patterns and routine change. Late nights combined with alcohol, late breakfasts and caffeine withdrawal are common factors. Lack of sleep for other reasons such as depression, exam pressure or menopausal hot flushes are also triggers.
- Environment – loud noise, smoke, bright or flickering lights, strong smells (especially chemical smells or perfume) and work environment.
- Travel – associated triggers include lack of sleep, stress of preparations, missed meals, dehydration, change to routine and crossing time zones. We don't know whether oxygen and pressure changes in aircraft cabins specifically trigger attacks, but loud engine noise, cramped seats and the smell of perfume in the duty-free shop certainly don't help!
- Weather – changes in barometric pressure during thunderstorms can be associated with increased migraine frequency, but data are conflicting. Humidity and bright sunlight can trigger attacks.
- Hormones – natural hormone changes occurring during menstruation, pregnancy or menopause, or those from using the pill or hormone replacement therapy are triggers for migraine in some women.
- Exertion – this can bring on a migraine, or more usually makes it worse. It can include exercise, sexual activity, coughing, sneezing or straining on the toilet. If you have migraine or any headache associated with exertion, you should discuss this with your doctor to confirm the diagnosis. It is mostly not a reason for concern, but underlying causes should be excluded.
- Emotion – the mechanisms are unclear, but any emotion (e.g. stress, anger or even excitement) can be a trigger. You may get through the stressful time and get the migraine on relaxation afterward.

- Other illnesses – untreated or uncontrolled illnesses (e.g. coughs, colds and flu, or eye, sinus, jaw, teeth or neck problems) may trigger migraine.

Migraine and other medical conditions

There is an association between migraine and other illnesses, including depression, anxiety, epilepsy and vertigo. This does not mean that having migraine causes these conditions; it is just that they are more likely to affect people who also have migraine. We need research to understand these connections. It may be more than a coincidence that anti-depressant and anti-epileptic medications can be very effective migraine preventatives, even if you don't have depression or epilepsy. Other medical conditions may influence the migraine medications prescribed by your doctor. If you have depression, then your migraine medication might help both conditions at the same time. If your depression improves then the migraine could too.

Migraine with aura is a marker for being at a higher risk for stroke and, in women, for heart disease. The connection is less clear if you do not have migraine aura. A recent study also suggested that people with migraine with aura are more likely to have 'white matter lesions'. These small areas of altered brain tissue can show up on brain scans, but there are no obvious symptoms. We don't know whether these are significant and research is ongoing.

There isn't much you can do about the tendency to migraine with aura, so don't be overly concerned. You'll already be trying to reduce attacks and this could reduce any risk, although significance of migraine frequency is unknown. It makes sense to concentrate on what you can do to reduce the risks for stroke and heart disease. This means giving up smoking, maintaining a healthy weight and, for women, not using combined hormonal contraceptives. Also have your blood pressure and cholesterol checked regularly and treated if necessary.

Having migraine might actually protect you from some diseases too! Although further work is required, recent research suggested that women with migraine are about 30 per cent less likely to develop breast cancer.

Does migraine improve?

There is currently discussion about migraine being a progressive condition, in which changes in the central nervous system may cause a few people to develop frequent migraine attacks more readily. We need more research in this area. Fortunately, for most people who do not over-use their medications, migraine is an episodic disorder. Frequency of attacks varies considerably over a life time. You can have gaps of weeks, months or even years at various stages in your life. Migraine can be worse for women when their hormones change as they approach the menopause.

Usually, for both men and women, migraine generally improves with age. Migraine attacks tend to become both less frequent and less severe. Don't wish your life away though! Migraine isn't guaranteed to disappear, and you must always do what you can to reduce the frequency of attacks.

3

Migraine: coping with medication

Symptomatic (acute) medications are used to treat migraine symptoms of head pain and nausea when they occur. When you treat a migraine attack, try to use the right drug, at the right dose and at the right time. This gives it the best chance of working. This chapter outlines how to make the right choice of medication and suggests a simple two-step strategy to treat a migraine attack. It also considers preventatives, taken daily.

Some medications are purchased over-the-counter and others are only obtained on prescription. Not all suit everyone because of side effects, especially at higher doses or if you have other medical conditions. Always read the packet insert information carefully. If your medication is not working or you have concerns about how it is affecting you, then see your doctor or pharmacist.

Medications for migraine symptoms

The right drug is the one that works best for you, with a minimum of side effects. Recommended medications for migraine symptoms in adults are as follows.

Simple painkillers

These are available over-the-counter. Try aspirin 600–900 milligrams (mg; two to three tablets) to start. You can repeat the dose every four to six hours, to a maximum of four grams over 24 hours. A good alternative is ibuprofen 400–600 mg (two to three tablets) to start, then repeated every four to six hours to a maximum of 2.4 grams per day. Paracetamol 1000 mg (two tablets) is well tolerated and works for some people, but it is less effective than aspirin or ibuprofen for migraine. It can be repeated every four to six hours to a maximum of four grams in 24 hours.

Anti-sickness (anti-emetic) drugs

Anti-sickness drugs help with nausea and vomiting. Some of them (e.g. domperidone and metoclopramide) also have a 'pro-kinetic' activity.

The stomach and gut shuts down during a migraine attack meaning treatments taken by mouth may not work well. By keeping everything moving, the addition of an anti-emetic can encourage rapid absorption of your painkiller or triptan. It is worth taking these drugs even if you don't feel sick early in your attack. Try a domperidone tablet (10 mg) at the onset. You can buy this over-the-counter. An alternative is a domperidone suppository, which can be prescribed by your doctor. Repeat doses (up to maximum daily limits) during the migraine attack to help other tablets to work and ease nausea and vomiting, if you have these symptoms.

Non-steroidal anti-inflammatory drugs

Non-steroidal anti-inflammatory drugs (NSAIDs) include naproxen tablets, diclofenac tablets or diclofenac suppositories. NSAIDs can cause stomach irritation, so additional protective medication may also be prescribed.

Triptans

These are a specific type of anti-migraine drug. They can alleviate headache and all associated migraine symptoms. They are discussed in more detail below.

Migraine medications to avoid

Using the right treatments means avoiding the wrong ones! These include morphine, pethidine, dihydrocodeine and combination painkillers that contain caffeine and codeine. These help other pain conditions, but when they are used to treat migraine they can make you feel more sick, cause your gut to shut down even further and be addictive.

Two steps to treat migraine

This is a two-step strategy to treat a migraine attack in adults. The first step may be sufficient, and the medications needed can be bought over-the-counter. If step one doesn't work, then proceed to step two, for which you will need a prescription from your doctor.

Step one

- At the start of a migraine when the head pain is mild, take a *soluble* preparation of your preferred simple painkiller.

- Combine this with an anti-sickness medication. This will help with any sickness, but importantly it will help painkillers to work better.
- Repeat doses as necessary, according to the packet instructions. Repeat the anti-sickness medication to help the painkillers to work, even if you don't feel sick.

If step one has not worked within an hour, then proceed to step two.

Step two

- Take your preferred triptan or an NSAID such as diclofenac, as prescribed by your doctor.
- Combine this with an anti-sickness medication. This will help with any sickness, but importantly it will help the triptans or NSAIDs to work better.
- Repeat doses as necessary but without exceeding the maximum daily dose allowed for the medication type.

If a moderate or severe migraine attack is present when you wake or if you always need to proceed to step two, then start with step two and miss out step one.

Treat symptoms early

The right time to treat your migraine attack is as early as possible. Clinical trials suggest that treating an attack when the head pain is mild works best. It is important to distinguish between migraine and a mild tension-type headache (TTH); otherwise you could be treating headaches that might go away anyway. Keep treatments near so that they are convenient when you need them quickly.

Get the dose right

The right dose is high enough to work well for you but with the fewest side effects. You may need to try different starting doses. Generally, use higher doses at the beginning of an attack and repeat as necessary. One aspirin (300 mg) might not do anything, but three (900 mg) could be enough to stop a migraine at its onset.

It is not a problem to use high doses over a few days (within the maximum daily limits and in the absence of troublesome side effects) if you are treating migraine infrequently, such as once a month. If you are treating migraines most weeks, then you might be at risk for side effects and medication over-use, and a preventative may be more helpful.

Remember – it is not the doses that are important but the number of days treated. Don't use triptans or combination tablets for more than ten days in a month or painkillers for more than 15 days in a month.

Find a medication type to suit you

Medication should ideally get into your blood stream quickly. If you are feeling or being sick and your stomach and gut are shutting down, this can be difficult. Different formulations of medications are available to help. There are tablets, mouth dispersible preparations, suppositories, injections and nasal sprays. You may need to experiment to find what suits you best.

Try to use the soluble painkillers or ones that dissolve on your tongue, which are more rapidly absorbed. Dissolve them in a sweet fizzy drink to help absorption and give your blood sugar level a boost.

NSAIDs such as diclofenac and anti-sickness medications such as domperidone are available as suppositories. You insert these small pellets into your back passage (rectum), where they are absorbed rapidly into your blood stream. They are worth trying because they are highly effective, especially if you feel nauseous or vomit early in attacks, making tablets difficult to use.

Triptans – specific anti-migraine drugs

Triptans are a class of anti-migraine drugs that work on serotonin receptors in the brain. Clinical trials have shown that they are all effective at stopping migraine symptoms. Milligram dosages vary between the different triptans and cannot be compared. It is finding one that works well for you that is important.

The first triptan developed, sumatriptan, is now available over-the-counter (50 mg tablet) if you complete a form checked by the pharmacist. The other triptans and different formulations of sumatriptan are only available on prescription.

Types of triptans available

There are seven different triptans available in the UK. Some are in different formulations making them more convenient to take. The formulations available are as follows:

- tablets (almotriptan 12.5 mg, eletriptan 20 mg and 40 mg, frovatriptan 2.5 mg, naratriptan 2.5 mg, sumatriptan 50 mg and 100 mg, rizatriptan 5 mg and 10 mg and zolmitriptan 2.5 mg);

- mouth dispersible, which dissolve in the mouth and do not require water (rizatriptan 10 mg and zolmitriptan 2.5 mg and 5 mg);
- nasal sprays (sumatriptan 20 mg and zolmitriptan 5 mg); and
- injection, provided in a preloaded auto-injector device for simple self-use (sumatriptan 6 mg).

Side effects of triptans

Side effects include a feeling of throat and chest tightness or pressure, nausea, tiredness and a heavy sensation in the limbs. Some side effects are difficult to distinguish from migraine symptoms, but if one triptan does not appear to agree with you then another might. The chest pressure symptoms in otherwise healthy people are not a cause for concern unless you feel pain rather than pressure. If you develop pain having not experienced it before with your usual triptan, then seek medical advice.

Triptans are not recommended for children, those over 65 or pregnant women. If you are at risk for heart disease or stroke or had these in the past, you will not be able to use triptans because they constrict blood vessels. You may be able to use triptans if you have had high blood pressure, but only if it is well controlled by medication.

Relapse with triptans

Relapse is when a migraine attack initially responds to a triptan but returns within 48 hours. A second dose is usually effective, but relapse can continue over several days. If relapse occurs repeatedly when treating your migraine, then discuss changing the triptan with your doctor. Combining triptans with NSAIDs and an anti-sickness medication at the start of an attack may be helpful.

Tips for using triptans

The triptan your doctor prescribes may depend on other medications that you are currently taking, because triptans can interact with some antibiotics, blood pressure tablets and anti-depressants.

- Take triptans with or without food, except rizatriptan, which should be used on an empty stomach.
- Use your triptan at the onset of migraine headache. They don't work if they are used during the aura phase of a migraine attack.
- Only use your triptan when you know that the headache is a migraine.

- Repeat the starting dose after two hours if the migraine goes away and comes back. Don't repeat if the first dose did not work. With the exception of zolmitriptan, which can be repeated after two hours, research shows second doses are unlikely to work.
- If your usual starting dose of a triptan is not effective, your doctor may suggest a higher starting dose. This can increase side effects and is not recommended for all triptans.
- Try a triptan for at least three separate migraine attacks when you have been free of migraine for at least a week. Sometimes an individual migraine might not respond, so it is worth trying again.
- If a triptan does not work or has side effects, try an alternative (or the same one in a different formulation) because another one may be effective.
- If the triptan needs to work very quickly or if nausea and vomiting are a problem, then your doctor may consider zolmitriptan nasal spray or sumatriptan injection.

Medications for migraine prevention

A preventative (prophylactic) medication is one that you take every day to reduce the number of migraine attacks. Used in addition to pain-killers or triptans for migraine symptoms, research evidence suggests that the following drugs can be useful preventatives.

Beta-blockers

These drugs are commonly prescribed for treatment of high blood pressure and angina. They are not suitable if you have certain medical conditions, including asthma. A course of propanolol twice daily can be helpful to prevent migraine. Metoprolol or atenolol are also used, and it is worth trying a different beta-blocker if one is not effective. Side effects are tiredness, cold feet and hands, and dizziness.

Amitriptyline

Amitriptyline is a tricyclic anti-depressant that can help to prevent migraine, particularly if you also have TTH, other pain conditions or disturbed sleep. Note that your doctor does not think you are depressed if he or she suggests this medication. More information on amitriptyline is available in Chapter 7.

Anti-epileptic drugs (or neuromodulators)

These are used at lower doses than for epilepsy control. They are not recommended during pregnancy, and so adequate contraception is advised. Clinical trials have shown that topiramate once or twice daily can help to prevent migraine attacks. The doses are built up gradually. Side effects of topiramate include pins and needles, weight loss and changes in mood, which usually settle with continued use. Sodium valproate twice daily can also be helpful; its side effects include nausea, tiredness, weight gain and hair loss. There is less evidence that gabapentin is effective. Side effects of gabapentin include dizziness and sedation.

Methysergide

Methysergide three times daily is licensed for use in migraine and cluster headache prevention, and it is very effective for both. It is used by specialists if other treatments have not been successful. See Chapter 9 for optimal use to avoid potential side effects.

Other drugs

Other drugs such as pizotifen and clonidine have been used for migraine prevention, but the drugs mentioned above are more effective.

Why use a preventative?

Preventative medications don't cure migraine, but they are useful if you have frequent migraines because they can reduce the number of attacks by up to half. They can also help if migraines are severe and disabling or if they don't respond well to symptomatic treatments, even if they are not very frequent. Regularly losing two or more days a month to severe attacks can prompt consideration of preventative treatment.

If your migraines always respond to treatment for symptoms, then preventatives may not be necessary. If your migraines have increased and you are using symptomatic medication on two or three days each week, then you are at risk of developing a medication over-use headache. A short course of a preventative could be enough to break the cycle.

How long to use preventatives

If the medication works well, then the plan is not for you to stay on daily preventatives indefinitely, although some people do remain on them for long periods. Headache specialists usually recommend that you stay on the effective dose for about six months and then gradually reduce the dose over two or three weeks. If migraine returns during this time, then the dose can be increased again. Typically, when you stop preventative medication the improvement is maintained.

If a preventative does not appear to be working, it is best to continue for a minimum of two to three months at the required dose to give it the best chance of success. The only reason to give up is unacceptable side effects. These can sometimes be reduced by lowering the dose for a while and waiting before increasing again. If you have given the preventative a proper trial and it doesn't work, then your doctor can usually suggest alternatives.

Tips for using preventatives

Although none of us wants to take tablets every day, sometimes a short course can break the cycle of troublesome migraine. Here are some tips.

- You should feel willing and motivated to use medication daily. If you keep forgetting or changing your mind, then it won't have a chance to work properly.
- Discuss with your doctor why you need to take the medication and what to expect. The choices might be influenced by other medical conditions.
- Usually, doses are built up slowly to give your body a chance to get used to the medication. If you follow the instructions carefully, you are less likely to get troublesome side effects. This slow dose increase can mean that medication takes longer to start working. This can be two to four weeks, and so you do have to be patient.
- Remember not to give up too soon, especially if you experience side effects – they are often transient.
- Keep a diary to assess whether treatment is working. Sometimes it isn't the frequency of the migraine that improves, but the severity, duration or even the response to symptomatic treatments.

4

Migraine: coping strategies and other treatment options

Apart from using medications, how else can you cope? Having a healthy lifestyle and a positive approach can really make a difference, and we look at this in the last chapters of the book. This chapter focuses on understanding migraine triggers and your migraine threshold. It also outlines potential new treatment options, such as surgery for migraine.

Identifying migraine triggers

You may be able to identify your migraine triggers by keeping a diary or by thinking about factors that led to an attack during the two or three days beforehand. You might have recognized the migraine triggers listed in Chapter 2 or found that that none seem particularly relevant. Disappointingly, that is the nature of migraine triggers. They are different for everyone, and even your identified triggers won't be the same for every attack, because their effects are not always predictable.

Understanding migraine triggers

It would make coping with migraine so much easier if it were as simple as avoiding known triggers. However, we don't understand how triggers work. It appears that people with migraine react in an over-sensitive way to environmental or chemical triggers such as loud noise, bright lights or specific foods. Triggers may work directly to cause migraine attacks, but not necessarily. Exposure to a trigger can mean a migraine at one time but not at others. This is because triggers work together in more complicated ways to cause migraine attacks and to affect your threshold for developing them.

Trigger factors and warning symptoms

Prodromes or warning symptoms of a migraine are easily mistaken for triggers in the early stages of an attack, before the headache begins. You crave chocolate, the migraine begins and chocolate is regarded as the trigger. Actually, the food craving was a warning of an attack that had already begun. Likewise, over-activity can be regarded as a trigger, when your behaviour change was really a pre-headache symptom.

Recognizing what might be happening with triggers and prodromes is important. If you can have something to eat and drink at this stage, perhaps have a lie down or at least a few minutes to relax, then you may be able to stop an attack developing. If the migraine headache does begin, then ensure that you have your medication ready to treat it early.

Your migraine threshold

The threshold theory of migraine is a useful way of thinking about migraine triggers. Your threshold is the level at which there are sufficient triggering influences of any kind to provoke a migraine attack. At the City of London Migraine Clinic we ask patients to think of *how many* triggers they need to start a migraine attack, rather than which one might cause it.

Imagine a ladder of triggers. With each trigger you climb up a rung of the ladder. Once you reach a certain level you cross your threshold and develop a migraine attack. For example, you may be tired, have a stressful day at work, not drink enough water *and* have your lunch late. On their own, these triggers might not have started an attack, but together they add up to tip you over your threshold.

Raising and lowering the migraine threshold

Your individual migraine threshold is determined by your genes and your tendency to have migraine. This means that people who are prone to frequent migraine have lower thresholds for developing attacks – that is, they have fewer rungs of the trigger ladder to climb.

The threshold for developing a migraine attack may be made higher by taking daily preventative drugs. This could mean that you need more triggers to get an attack.

Triggers such as illness or a menstrual period in women can act in two ways. They may act directly to cause a migraine attack but they can also have the effect of lowering your threshold so that other triggers are more likely to provoke an attack. Stress, late nights or a glass of wine can trigger a migraine in a woman at period time, but at other times these same triggers don't provoke an attack.

By recognizing how triggers can build up, you may be able to do something about the trigger that actually tips you over the threshold.

This is especially if you think that triggers might be working to lower your threshold. These principles work for me and are an important part of how I cope with my own migraine. It is now rare that I have a migraine attack without knowing why. I know that at times of stress, tiredness or ill health I have to drink plenty, eat regularly and make allowances. Otherwise, I will almost certainly get a migraine attack.

Coping with triggers for migraine

Not all attacks have an obvious cause, and you cannot avoid triggers all of the time. Don't allow triggers to become an additional worry. See if you can identify what, if anything, is a trigger for you. Triggers are important, but not necessarily significant for everyone, because they do not just 'turn on' an attack. The most important thing is to work out what is relevant for you. If you cannot identify triggers then don't be overly concerned – some of them you can't do much about anyway. Only avoid triggers if you notice a pattern. Otherwise, it is too easy to start avoiding favourite foods (such as chocolate), an alcoholic drink or evenings out with friends. Life can then become rather dreary and you feel that you are really missing out – all because of migraine!

If you want to eliminate a suspected trigger, then do so systematically. Keep a diary to see whether it really makes a difference and just change one thing at a time. Small changes are much more manageable anyway.

As a migraineur you must recognize that you may be very sensitive, but don't become a slave to trigger avoidance.

Lifestyle trigger factors

Try to make sure that your lifestyle prevents your migraine and does not trigger attacks. These are the trigger factors over which you have most control.

- Diet – eat regularly and don't miss meals.
- Fluids – drink at least two litres of water throughout the day.
- Sleep – get into a regular sleep pattern and make sure that you get enough rest. Try to maintain it at weekends and when you are out of your routine, such as holidays.
- Exercise – get active and exercise regularly. Keep hydrated and eat regularly to keep blood sugar levels stable.

Environmental trigger factors

You may have little control over your environment, so concentrate on the factors that you can do something about.

- Noise, smoke and strong smells – these are sometimes difficult to avoid, but leave the environment if you recognize a trigger. If you have to be exposed to triggers (e.g. going to a loud concert), then get some early nights beforehand, remember to eat regularly and keep drinking water.
- Weather – although you can't change the weather, you can avoid other triggers such as dehydration if the weather is humid. A large sun hat and sunglasses can help if bright sunlight is a trigger.
- Travel – it is impossible to avoid some potential triggers when travelling, but minimize those you can. Get enough sleep and break up journeys if possible. Ensure that you eat regularly and keep hydrated – remember that air travel is very dehydrating. Avoid alcohol while flying, because its effect is more potent. Be organized in your preparations and allow plenty of time so that travelling is no more stressful that it needs to be.
- Visual stress – if bright or flickering lights from the TV, computer screens or school whiteboards are triggers, then take regular breaks from the screen, try to avoid tension build-up in your neck and shoulders, and keep hydrated. There has been concern about compact fluorescent integrated light bulbs causing migraine. Newer bulbs are now supposed to emit a constant flicker-free light and no longer emit the blue light that some migraineurs are sensitive to.
- Work environment – work brings many migraine triggers. Poor lighting, ventilation, shift patterns, over-time, poor ergonomics at your computer workstation, no regular meal breaks, impossible management targets, telephones and computers are just a few. Poor posture can cause muscle strain. Identify whether these could be making your migraine worse. Regular breaks and a few small changes may make a difference.

Psychological trigger factors

These can play an important role in migraine.

- Stress – this is often impossible to avoid. However, notice the impact that stress has on the other migraine triggers, such as missing meals and sleep. It lowers your migraine threshold so that other triggers more quickly build up to an attack. Avoid stress where you can. Regular breaks and time for hobbies and relaxation are important.

- Other emotions – anger, excitement and relaxation after stress are also difficult to avoid. Try to prevent controllable triggers from building up to cross your migraine threshold.

Hormonal trigger factors

Natural hormone changes can be significant triggers for migraine, or alter the threshold for getting them, at various stages in a woman's life.

Other illnesses

Get illnesses treated. Any illness can act as a trigger or lower your threshold for developing a migraine attack.

Rachael, 20

Rachael is a police officer. She shares a flat with friends. She has had migraine with aura since she was 18. Rachael remembers the first attack very clearly because it occurred after an important police examination.

On the bus home Rachael noticed an odd zigzag pattern of shimmering light in her left eye. It moved across from left to right and lasted for about 15 minutes. Rachael had felt tired after her examination, but by the time she arrived home she was feeling sick. She then developed an extremely severe headache. It was on one side of her temple and it pounded. She recalls being violently sick and then going to bed. Her flatmates were concerned because her face was so white. The next morning the headache was gone, but it was another few days until she felt well again.

The police occupational health doctor diagnosed the headache as migraine with aura. Rachael has had several similar episodes, with and without the visual symptoms of migraine aura. Rachael was advised that she should not use the combined oral contraceptive pill because of a slight increased risk for stroke in young women who also have migraine aura. She was prescribed a triptan to take at the start of a migraine headache. Rachael visited us at the City of London Migraine Clinic because she felt that her medication no longer worked and she wanted further advice. Her migraine attacks had increased in frequency and her senior officers were concerned about her having to go off duty.

The specialist confirmed typical migraine with and without aura and recommended a triptan nasal spray. This would be quick and easy to take on duty at the onset of the head pain, after the aura phase. If possible, the addition of an anti-sickness drug like domperidone would help with the sickness and with absorption of the triptan, because even nasal sprays are mostly absorbed from the gut.

The doctor discussed why Rachael's migraine attacks might have increased. She was currently on a new work placement that meant that she was working irregular hours. The shift patterns had affected her sleep, and meal breaks on duty were often many hours apart. Although Rachael could do little about the shifts, she was told to try to drink plenty of water, cut down her ten coffees a day and to eat regularly, taking snacks with her if necessary. She was also encouraged to eat more proper meals when she was off duty, because she admitted to living on takeaway food with her flatmates. Rachael needed more time for relaxing too. The new post was demanding, and Rachael said that she sometimes spent her days off just catching up on sleep. She never felt refreshed. It was suggested that she should keep to a regular sleep pattern, even on her time off.

At her follow-up visit Rachael had kept migraine diaries, which showed significant improvement. The nasal spray and anti-sickness combination worked quickly and effectively. Importantly for her, Rachael was able to continue working during an attack. The diary showed that she should try to take her medications as early as possible when the head pain started, including migraine attacks without aura. Early treatment would mean that any attack would be less likely to develop.

It had been difficult to eat regularly and drink enough water, but it had become part of Rachael's routine and she thought it helped. She had also tried to improve her overall diet and go to for a run on her days off. This was enjoyable and relaxing. It gave her more energy rather than less and she slept better too. Rachael felt more positive about coping with her migraine. She was more confident managing with her new treatments, and the small changes she made in her lifestyle had helped make her attacks less frequent.

New treatment options for migraine

In recent years various exciting new strategies for migraine prevention have been introduced. However, at the time of writing none of the following strategies has been shown in research studies to be consistently safe and effective, and as a result they are not widely available. These approaches are usually only considered if standard treatments have failed. Migraine Action and the Migraine Trust can advise on recent developments. (See Useful addresses at the end of this book.)

Hole in the heart closure

Recent research did not demonstrate that closure of a hole in the heart (patent foramen ovale – PFO) is better at preventing migraine than standard preventative drug treatments. Because people with migraine with aura are around twice as likely to have a PFO, trials are continuing to see whether closure can help. Currently, headache specialists do not recommend this procedure for migraine outside of clinical trials, because it is invasive and not without risk.

PFO affects around a quarter of the general population. It occurs when the opening between the upper chambers of the heart (atria) fail to close completely at birth. Although most people do not suffer any ill effects, heart specialists may recommend PFO closure for medical reasons. This can be done under anaesthesia and involves the insertion of a small device into a large vein in the groin. This is then passed up into the heart and positioned to close the PFO.

Some people who have had their PFOs closed have found coincidentally that their migraines have improved. Therefore, recent research has been done to find out whether this procedure should be undertaken specifically for migraine prevention. The link is only with migraine with aura and we don't know why – it could be genetic. The mechanisms are unclear. Blood that goes through the opening has not been filtered by the lungs, and it is possible that it contains tiny particles or chemicals that reach the brain and could trigger the onset of migraine aura.

Botulinum toxin injection

Botulinum toxin is a neurotoxin that paralyses muscles. It has been used in medicine to help movement disorders and muscle spasms. In the cosmetic industry relaxation of the facial muscles can help reduce the appearance of wrinkles and frown lines. Considerable recent interest focuses on whether botulinum toxin can help with tension-type headache (TTH) and migraine because of its effect on muscles and on sensory nerve function.

Botulinum toxin is administered in a series of tiny injections into muscles in the head and neck area. The effects are short lasting and treatment needs repeating. It is usually well tolerated with minimal side effects. Clinical trials so far have not provided clear evidence that botulinum toxin works for headaches, and we need more good quality research studies. Therefore, this treatment is not widely recommended by headache specialists.

Greater occipital nerve injection

Greater occipital nerve injections are used at some specialist centres for migraine, cluster headache and TTH. The greater occipital nerve is at the back of the head. By injections of local anaesthetic and steroids, pain transmission along the nerve can be blocked. Pain relief can last for several months. The injections can be repeated and side effects (including dizziness and slight hair loss at the injection site) are minimal. Ongoing research will show whether this treatment works.

Migraine and surgery

Surgical techniques such as deep brain stimulation and continuous stimulation of the occipital nerve via electrode have been used for cluster headache. They have been carried out in severe migraine cases under clinical trial conditions.

Currently, all surgery for migraine is experimental. This includes any surgical manipulation of muscles, blood vessels or nerves in the head and face. We need more detailed, large-scale research studies, which will provide both short-term and long-term safety data and evidence about whether any improvement is maintained.

If you have severe migraine and/or other headaches, you may consider surgery in the hope of finding relief from your pain. This always needs to be carefully considered, because surgery and anaesthesia carry risks that need to be weighed up against any potential benefits. No surgical techniques have yet been shown to help migraine better than standard available treatments.

Tips for coping with migraine

- Identify migraine triggers that you can do something about and deal with them. Don't worry about those you can't change.
- Think about *all* aspects of your life, including home, work and leisure.
- Don't underestimate small changes.
- Remember the trigger ladder.
- Despite optimal trigger management, always be prepared if a migraine breaks through.
- Keep informed about new developments in migraine. New treatments and medications are being developed.

5

Migraine in children and older people

Primarily a disorder of men and women during mid-life, migraine frequently occurs in children, although it can take different forms. Many people grow out of migraine as they get older, particularly women after the menopause.

Migraine in children

Migraine occurs in children and teenagers, particularly if it runs in the family. It affects about ten per cent of children aged between five and 15. Migraine in children should always be assessed by a doctor. This is essential in children under 12 with a new headache, new symptoms or a fever. There is not usually anything else wrong, but other causes must be excluded. Brain tumours are rare and, as for adults, headaches are not usually the only symptom.

Typically, migraine in children tends to be shorter lasting than in adults – perhaps only one or two hours. The headache can be on both sides of the head, and severe vomiting is often a feature. Migraine aura may also be present. Children are good at drawing what they see during their aura, which can help to confirm the diagnosis! Aura may disappear in adulthood migraine and come back in later life without a headache. Migraine often recedes during teenage years to return during the twenties.

Abdominal migraine and childhood periodic syndromes

In young children under 12, head pain may not be the main problem. Children can complain of intermittent general stomach pain that may or may not be accompanied by nausea and vomiting. This is called abdominal migraine and it can reoccur in attacks like migraine.

Other 'childhood periodic syndromes' of recurring symptoms are marked by the child being completely well between episodes. Symptoms may include nausea, vomiting, vertigo and tilting of the neck. Children don't have a headache, but they can be very pale and sensitive to light and sound. A doctor must always diagnose these syndromes because many other conditions such as bowel disorders and infections can give rise to similar symptoms. These syndromes are related to migraine in adults, and around half of young children will go on to develop typical migraine in adulthood.

Coping with migraine in children

Coping with migraine in children means involving them in their care as much as possible, as appropriate for their age. Even young children are often very good at keeping detailed (and beautifully illustrated) diaries when requested. This can help to identify avoidable triggers. In children these frequently include the following:

- not eating regularly (or enough, especially during a growth spurt),
- exercise,
- lack of fluids,
- irregular sleeping patterns,
- exposure to flickering lights,
- over-excitement,
- travel and
- stress at school or home.

Most children do not require medication for migraine attacks, which tend to be short lasting. Severe vomiting may mean that tablets can't be taken anyway. If symptom treatments are required, these are usually ibuprofen (aspirin should not be taken by under-16s) or domperidone for sickness and nausea. None of the triptans are licensed for use in under-18s apart from sumatriptan nasal spray for adolescents aged 12–17 years. All medications should be discussed with the child's doctor, because not all are suitable for children and doses may need adjusting according to weight and height of the child. Medication over-use headache occurs in children and teenagers as well as adults. If simple strategies are not effective then a child should be assessed by a specialist children's doctor (a paediatrician) with an interest in headache.

Migraine can be disabling in children and mean frequent time lost from school. If necessary, parents should seek help for migraine in a child, because it can be a source of family stress. Often it is the parents who need most reassurance!

Take time to inform your child's school about their migraine. The school may not be sympathetic unless they understand how migraine affects the child and how they can help. Fluids and a lie down in the first aid room may be enough to stop an attack developing. At home it is very important to maintain regular routines for sleeping, eating, getting up and getting dressed, homework and time on the computer. Try not to let migraine dominate your child's life. If possible they should be strongly encouraged to continue all the activities they enjoy, such as sport, hobbies and seeing their friends.

Migraine in older people

If you are not lucky enough to grow out of migraine, like the majority, this doesn't mean that there is anything wrong with you. Generally, though, migraine attacks are less severe with fewer accompanying symptoms as you get older. Some people who have had migraine with aura find that they experience the aura without a headache as they get older. You should discuss this with your doctor, to exclude the possibility of stroke or transient ischaemic attack, which are more common with advancing age as arteries fur up.

Migraine rarely develops for the first time in someone over 50, so your doctor will usually look for other causes for headache. These include dental issues, jaw and neck problems, facial pains (trigeminal neuralgia) and inflammation of the arteries (temporal arteritis).

Coping with migraine in older people

If troublesome migraines persist then you will need to take extra care to try to reduce attacks and treat them appropriately. This means eating enough, drinking plenty of fluids and avoiding over-using medications to treat migraines. You should chat with your doctor if you have any concerns, your headache changes, you develop a new headache or symptoms, or you have other medical problems.

Various factors can adversely influence migraine in later life. Ill-fitting dentures make proper nutrition difficult, and resulting unstable blood sugar levels could trigger migraine. Social isolation may contribute to depression and emotional triggers.

If you are on a tight budget and only heat one room using a gas appliance, you are at higher risk for carbon monoxide poisoning if the appliance is faulty. Headaches and nausea at home that improve outside in the fresh air are an early sign, although this warning does not always occur. Carbon monoxide poisoning from this odourless, colourless gas can cause unconsciousness and death. The flame should burn blue, not yellow, and there should be no soot deposits. Regular checking of appliances and fitting a carbon monoxide detector are important.

Having migraine does not appear to increase your risk of high blood pressure or cognitive impairment as you get older. However, migraine may more readily co-exist with these and other illnesses. These may impact on both the migraine itself and the treatments your doctor prescribes.

As you get older you are much more sensitive to the side effects of all medications, some of which can cause headaches. Ageing affects our blood vessels and causes our digestive, liver and kidney function to be less efficient. You and your doctor should watch out for side effects of all of your medications, including those for migraine. Sometimes doses need to be reduced or changed because of another medical condition. Manufacturers don't recommend the use of triptans in people over 65 because they can constrict diseased blood vessels in the heart. Your doctor or specialist may consider prescribing triptans 'off-label' for infrequent use if you are a healthy non-smoker with normal blood pressure.

6

Tension-type headache: causes and triggers

Tension-type headache (TTH) is a 'normal' kind of headache. The most common primary headache and usually successfully self-treated, it is little more than an occasional inconvenience. You only need help from healthcare professionals when headaches either increase in number or no longer respond to painkillers.

TTH has previously been known as tension headache, muscle contraction headache, stress headache, ordinary headache and psychogenic headache. These names give clues as to possible causes. Mild and often featureless, TTH lacks the distinguishing symptoms that characterize migraine or cluster headache. However, TTH can exist with other headaches and may be mistaken for migraine without aura. Recognition is important because, ideally, different headaches should be dealt with separately if management is to be successful.

Although usually less disabling than migraine, the low impact headache of TTH can still be a real nuisance. If TTH becomes chronic rather than episodic, it can have a severe impact on your life.

Symptoms of tension-type headache

Apart from a headache, you may notice no other symptoms with TTH. Pain may be pressing, tightening or squeezing. TTH is usually only mild or, at worst, moderate. It does not throb and tends to be on both sides of the head. This is unlike migraine, in which pain is severe, one-sided and pulsating. The pain can start from or spread into the neck. Tenderness in head and neck muscles may be noticed when pressed with the fingers.

TTH lasts anything from 30 minutes to seven days in the episodic form, but it is often just a few hours. Unlike migraine, the headache doesn't worsen with routine physical activities. You don't often have to stop what you are doing, but you may be aware that you are working less effectively. Nausea is not usually a problem, although there can be loss of appetite. There may be heightened sensitivity to loud noises and bright lights, which is one of the reasons why TTH can be confused with migraine.

Paul, 38
'I get a dull kind of pain like a tight band or vice around my head. It tends to come on in the later part of the day and my neck also feels stiff. I don't feel sick and I can carry on working. I take a couple of paracetamol and it goes. I'm a bus driver and I don't think that sitting all day helps. Recently, I've started swimming twice a week and I think that eases the tension in my neck.'

Different kinds of tension-type headache

There are three categories of TTH, based on how often the headache occurs. *Infrequent episodic TTH* occurs on average less than one day per month and has little impact on individuals. These are the kind of headaches that occur now and again and do not bother us too much.

The other two types, however, occur much more frequently and may require medical help. They can be very disabling and debilitating. *Frequent episodic TTH* occurs between one and 14 days per month for at least three months. TTH is classified as *chronic TTH* when it occurs on 15 or more days per month on average, for more than three months. Chronic TTH starts as episodic and in some people evolves over a period of time to the point at which pain becomes almost daily or even continuous. We do not know why this happens in some people and not others.

Who gets tension-type headache?

On average about half of adults have experienced an episodic TTH, but some studies suggest that this could be nearer 80 per cent. Chronic TTH is rare and affects about three per cent. TTH can occur at any age – including in children – but is most likely to occur in the forties, with women being more affected than men.

Causes of tension-type headache

TTH has not been well defined. Because it doesn't have any specific symptoms other than head pain, it has been difficult to quantify and research. Causes were previously considered psychological, but recent studies suggest a neurobiological basis (e.g. biology of the nerves involved in pain transmission and perception).

Although we are gaining new knowledge, underlying causes remain uncertain. We don't know whether the pain originates in the scalp and neck muscles and is referred (i.e. felt elsewhere), or whether there are disturbances in pain processing in the brain itself. It is possible that both mechanisms are important. Over-excitable nerve transmission from head and neck muscles may play a role in episodic TTH, and abnormalities in pain processing and generalized increased pain sensitivity could become important in chronic TTH when the headaches are more frequent.

Studies suggest an increased genetic risk for frequent episodic and chronic TTH, but not for infrequent episodic TTH.

Triggers for tension-type headache

Emotional tension and physical tension in scalp and neck muscles are the two main triggers associated with TTH. Mental tension and stress often, but not always, aggravate TTH. Also, people with frequent episodic and chronic TTH are more likely to be anxious and depressed than those with infrequent episodic TTH. Whether low mood is a cause or a result of the headaches is unknown. Physical tension and sometimes tenderness in the muscles of the scalp and neck are also implicated. These can occur from musculoskeletal abnormalities or for other reasons, such as poor posture or muscle strain (e.g. when lifting heavy objects or carrying heavy bags on a regular basis).

Josephine, 59
'I had a fall last year and broke my ankle. It took a long time to heal. I couldn't do the part time work I really enjoy which gets me out of the house. I remember feeling really low. I'd only ever had occasional headaches during my life, but at this time I seemed to be getting them once or twice a week. There were just a dull ache and didn't stop me from doing anything. I got even more fed up as they were just something else to deal with. My daughter suggested I told the GP [general practitioner] about them. He gave me a thorough check over, which was reassuring. He didn't prescribe anything, which I thought he might. He just said it was probably because I was much less mobile and not really myself. Once I got back to work, started moving again and feeling better, the headaches disappeared as quickly as they came. I hardly ever have one now.'

Does tension-type headache improve?

Episodic TTH often improves over time. In one recent study nearly half of adults with chronic and frequent episodic TTH were in remission at a three-year follow up. It is important to identify and treat any causes and additional problems such as migraine, medication over-use, musculoskeletal disorders, depression and sleep problems. This is because if these issues are not tackled first, then they may be underlying contributing factors to TTH. Unless they are properly managed, TTH is unlikely to respond well to any management strategy.

7

Coping with tension-type headache

Despite being an ordinary kind of headache, tension-type headache (TTH) can be a real blight on your life. If your headache responds to an occasional painkiller, then it is not too much of a problem. But what if the painkillers stop working or the headaches start happening frequently? In this chapter we look at ways in which you can help yourself and the treatments you can take.

Coping with tension-type headache without medical treatments

Although clinical studies don't show the benefit of particular non-drug management strategies on TTH, lifestyle changes can be worthwhile. Sometimes, keeping a diary and taking a step back to think about what could be influencing your headaches is revealing.

Simple coping strategies

If you feel a TTH developing, simple strategies (e.g. application of hot or cold packs) can be very soothing and surprisingly effective if done in the early stages. Massaging aching neck and shoulder muscles – even on yourself if there is no one to do it for you – can ease muscular tension.

Having something to eat or drink is always a good idea. Sometimes with vague kinds of headaches that are difficult to identify, it might just be a headache caused by hunger or dehydration.

Physical therapies

If you have musculoskeletal problems – particularly with your back, neck or shoulders – then physical therapies such as physiotherapy, osteopathy or chiropractic may be helpful. Make sure that your therapist is aware of your headaches in addition to any other problems, because this may influence their approach. Working with your therapist to improve your posture can also help TTH.

Complementary therapies

Some people report benefit with complementary therapies such as acupuncture and homeopathy.

Stress management

If you are feeling stressed as the headache is developing, try a change of environment; for instance, get away from your computer or out for a breath of fresh air. Because stress-related issues may play a role in TTH, any lifestyle changes to reduce stress may be helpful.

Exercise

TTH appears to be more common in sedentary people. Regular exercise can be beneficial.

Coping with tension-type headache using medical treatments

Drug treatments may be helpful, but in the long term it is better to identify and treat any underlying contributory factors first. These include muscular problems, sleep problems, depression or medication over-use.

Symptomatic (acute) drug treatments such as painkillers are appropriate for episodic TTH, occurring on no more than two days per week. More frequent use increases your chances of developing medication over-use headaches. Usually, no other treatments are needed. You can use maximum doses when the headache starts to stop it from developing. With episodic TTH this is normally all that is required, and the headache often responds to a single dose.

Frequent episodic or chronic TTH is a different matter. These often require prescription preventative drug treatments taken daily to gain relief from relentless headaches. Achieving this becomes much more difficult in longstanding chronic TTH. If medication has been overused, this must be recognized and tackled. Otherwise, it hinders headache diagnosis and stops any other treatment strategies from working properly.

Therefore treating chronic TTH with symptomatic treatments is not usually recommended. If you have frequent headaches you should see your doctor, who may prescribe a short course of the non-steroidal anti-inflammatory drug (NSAID) naproxen, taken regularly over a three-week period. This can break the cycle of frequent headaches and the habit of always reaching for painkillers.

If you have tried many different treatments, your doctor may refer you to a pain management clinic.

Medication for episodic tension-type headache symptoms

Clinical studies suggest that oral aspirin (600–900 milligrams [mg]) has the best effectiveness. Children under 16 should not use aspirin. Generally, the NSAIDs work well. Ibuprofen (400 mg) may be bought over-the-counter. Naproxen and diclofenac may be prescribed by a doctor. Stomach irritation and ulceration can sometimes be a side effect of all of these medications. Paracetamol (500–1000 mg) appears less effective but can be helpful for some, especially if other medications are not tolerated.

Opioids such as codeine or other strong analgesics and sedative hypnotics, including drugs like diazepam (Valium), are not recommended. This is because they make you drowsy and can be addictive.

Medication for prevention of tension-type headache

The best time to start preventatives is not clear, but because the risk of developing more headaches increases when they occur weekly, this may be the time to consider. If medication over-use with symptomatic treatments is occurring, then these treatments may have to be stopped before starting preventatives. It is not known whether preventatives can prevent or delay the transformation of episodic to chronic TTH that occurs in some people.

Amitriptyline

Amitriptyline is the treatment of choice, and there is evidence of its effectiveness in clinical studies. It is a tricyclic anti-depressant and is used in lower doses in TTH prevention than in depression. Your doctor prescribes it because it reduces pain and muscle tenderness and aids sleep, not because it is an antidepressant. If you are depressed, then your doctor will usually prescribe a newer type of anti-depressant.

Dose regimens for amitriptyline vary. You start with a low dose at night, gradually increasing at one-week to two-week intervals. The final dose will depend on when you feel benefit and how well you tolerate the drug. When improvement has been maintained for about six months, you can gradually reduce. It can be restarted if the headaches come back. The plan is usually to have a short course of the drug to break a headache cycle, not to stay on a daily drug for an indefinite period of time.

Side effects are typically minimal, provided doses are low and increases are gradual. Common side effects include dry mouth, constipation and blurred vision, but they usually improve with continued use. By taking amitriptyline two hours before bedtime, sedation the next day can be minimized. Remember that you can get side effects before the drug has started working, so it is important not to give up too soon. Amitriptyline can be very effective, so it is worth persevering for at least three months.

Other treatments

There is less evidence from clinical trials for TTH preventatives other than amitriptyline. Mirtazapine, alternative tricyclic antidepressants and tizanidine (a muscle relaxant) may be helpful. Clinical studies have not shown effectiveness for botulinum toxin injections into head and neck muscles.

Janice, 29

Janice is an accounts assistant for a large company. She attended the City of London Migraine Clinic because her headaches were increasingly frequent. Janice has always had the occasional headache, and two paracetamols usually resolved it fairly promptly. Now paracetamol had stopped working, so she no longer took it. The headaches were occurring up to four or five days a week. Janice is single, having split up with her boyfriend, who moved out of their flat. Janice is managing to pay the mortgage on her own but is finding it a struggle and is doing overtime to make ends meet.

Janice described the headaches as the same as she has always had, just more of them. The pain was mild and had more of a pressure quality rather than a throbbing or pulsating sensation. It spread from her neck and felt like a band of muscle tightness across the back of her head on both sides. Her neck muscles felt slightly tender. She didn't feel sick and had no other symptoms. Headaches could come on at any time of day and last from a couple of hours to all day. They didn't usually stop her from doing anything, but she felt that she was not performing as well at work as she could be.

After examining Janice and assessing her headache diary record card, the doctor diagnosed chronic TTH. This can sometimes evolve from an episodic form. In Janice's case this was not migraine, which can co-exist with TTH or be mistaken for it. Headaches due to over-using medication were excluded in Janice's case by the careful diary record that she kept. The doctor considered that Janice's stress with the break up of her relationship, coupled with extra hours of over-time spent mostly at a computer, contributed to increasing headaches. Janice agreed this was likely.

As Janice's headaches were frequent, not responding to medication and really troubling her, she started amitriptyline as a preventative to help with pain and muscle tenderness. Janice started at a low dose two hours before bedtime to minimize sedative effects the next day, and gradually increased the dose. She tolerated the medication well and, apart from a dry mouth and sleepiness at first, didn't notice any troublesome side effects. Janice was advised not to treat her headaches as they occurred unless she felt it was necessary, and in any case not on more than two days a week. Aspirin or ibuprofen was suggested. Janice did not feel that she could cut down her working hours because she needed the income, but she did agree to take more regular breaks from her computer, get advice about improving her posture and workstation set up, and try to get more exercise.

Janice was reassured that her headaches had no serious underlying cause. After six months Janice was able to stop taking the amitriptyline. Her headaches reduced rapidly because of the combination of preventative medication and more exercise in the form of swimming and a regular gym class. She still gets occasional headaches but these respond well to aspirin.

Tips for coping with tension-type headache

- If you are anxious about your headaches this can make them worse. Seek help if you need it.
- TTH can be difficult to recognize and co-exists with other headaches. Get a proper diagnosis if headaches are troublesome.
- Look after yourself and remember to eat and drink regularly.
- Keep a diary card to identify possible underlying factors.
- Focus on non-drug ways to cope and find new ways to relax and deal with stress.
- Get depression and anxiety treated. These make TTH worse and resistant to treatment.
- Become more active and do more exercise.
- Don't treat headaches on more than two or three days a week; otherwise a medication over-use headache may develop.

8

Cluster headache: causes and triggers

Jason, 35
'My worst ever experience. It is an excruciating, stabbing pain behind my right eye like a red-hot poker. I feel that my eye is being pushed out of my head. I can't sit still. I have to pace about. I scream and swear – I just can't help myself.'

Barbara, 42
'The pain is off the scale. The pain of every single attack is much, much worse than being in labour when I gave birth to my two children. Imagine giving birth four times a day and that might give you some idea of what I go through.'

These are some of the ways people with cluster headache have described their attacks. It is one of the most painful conditions known to mankind. In our City of London Migraine Clinic newsletter, Alan summed it up by telling us,

'It is difficult to describe the severity of the pain of cluster headache to those who have not experienced it. Imagine the pain if you slam your fingers in a door or hit your thumb with a hammer. Severe as the pain might be initially, it does not continue at that level of severity for long. The intense pain of a cluster headache is even worse and it can go on and on ... sometimes lasting for several hours.'

Recently, Sean confided to me,

'If you put ten of us having a cluster headache attack in the same room as a shotgun, we would all be tempted ... I would not be surprised if you opened the door to find at least one dead person ...'

No wonder that cluster headache is called 'suicide headache'. This isn't an exaggeration, because some people have been driven to take their lives. It is hard to imagine their pain and the total despair.

Cluster headache is a primary headache and, although it may co-exist with migraine, it requires specific diagnosis and treatment. Sometimes people say they have 'cluster migraines'. Certainly, during a bad run migraine days can group together, but cluster headache is a separate kind of headache.

Although it has distinctive features in its typical form, cluster headache is not always recognized. In the past it could take up to ten years for a proper diagnosis to be made! If you (or someone you know) may have cluster headache, it is important to get medical advice and access to effective treatments. Over-the-counter painkillers and self-help treatments are of no value in this incredibly severe headache.

Features of cluster headache

These vary from person to person and even attack to attack. You may not have every feature every time, but here are some of the main ones.

Intense, excruciating pain

This is felt on one side of your head only. Pain is never mild. It is often on the right side but can vary between attacks. It usually occurs in and around your eye. Sometimes it moves from behind your eye, feeling as though the eye itself is being pushed out. It can be in the temple region or spread to another part of the head. Pain feels like stabbing or boring like a knife, rather than having a throbbing quality. Pain comes on quickly with no warning and peaks within a matter of minutes. There is no gradual worsening, as seen with other types of headaches.

Intermittent, short pain attacks

These last between 15 minutes and three hours, if they are untreated. This is relatively short compared with migraine pain, which typically lasts 4–72 hours. They occur from once every other day to up to eight times a day. This can also happen at night, often waking you soon after falling asleep. It is easy to become exhausted.

Predictable attacks

The attacks often occur at exactly the same time each day or night. Likewise, bouts can start at the same time once or twice a year. Sometimes with the changing of the seasons, some people can also predict the onset of their bouts with amazing accuracy. How often they occur distinguishes the type of cluster headache you have.

One-sided accompanying symptoms

The symptoms occur just on the affected side of your head. This can seem very odd, but the other side is completely normal. Symptoms include a red eye, tears from the eye, a blocked or running nostril, and sweating and/or flushing on one side of the face or forehead. A smaller pupil, eyelid drooping and eyelid swelling can also occur on the affected side. They are difficult to observe on yourself. It may be your partner who notices changes during an attack, which can be minimal or quite marked and persist afterward. Symptoms such as nausea and light sensitivity associated with migraine are not typical in cluster headache, but they can occur. Sensitivity to light and sound may be just on the affected side. This is another difference from migraine.

Restless, agitated behaviour

Restless and agitated behaviour during an attack means you often cannot keep still. This is unlike migraine, in which the urge is to lie down. The need to pace about or rock back and forth can be uncontrollable. You may hold your head or bang it against the wall. Some people seek fresh or really cold air on their faces, which can help slightly. Severe pain can provoke unusually aggressive behaviour. Knowing that they cannot control themselves makes some people want to be left completely alone. You may not want to be touched or comforted, and this can be very difficult and disturbing for those trying to support you.

Neil, 43
'I have had clusters regularly twice a year for the past four years. They last for about six weeks. They always come around the same time in March and September. I never plan anything important at these times. I get about four attacks a day. Two of these are always during the night, and I always seem to get one about 3pm in the afternoon. My colleagues know that that they should just leave me alone, and we never plan a meeting for then!'

Types of cluster headache

The two types of cluster headache are distinguished by how often the headache attacks occur.

Episodic cluster headache

This affects about 80–90 per cent of people with cluster headache. Headache attacks cluster in episodic bouts lasting from two weeks to six months, with an average of about six to 12 weeks. The bouts of daily or near daily headaches occur two or three times a year. The onset may be at the same time each year and you know when it is coming. Sometimes there are gaps of several years between bouts.

Chronic cluster headache

This affects about 10–20 per cent of people with cluster headache. The cluster headache attacks don't have distinct bouts with pain-free gaps (remissions). Any remissions last less than a month and there is often no obvious pattern to your attacks. Episodic can evolve to chronic cluster headache in around ten per cent of people but we don't know why and it cannot be predicted. Chronic cluster headache is more difficult to treat and control than the episodic type. Fortunately, about 30 per cent of people with chronic cluster headache switch to the episodic type.

Who gets cluster headache?

Although cluster headache is rare, it still affects around three people per thousand in the UK. Cluster headache may be even more common but is under-diagnosed. Prevalence (the number of people who have it) in the UK is similar to that of multiple sclerosis, which is far more widely recognized. Anyone can develop cluster headache, including children, but it typically occurs between 20 and 40 years of age.

Unlike migraine and tension-type headache, cluster headache affects about five times more men than women. The proportion of women may be increasing. This could be due to better recognition, because women traditionally have been diagnosed with migraine instead. There is a type of headache similar to cluster headache that mainly affects women – paroxysmal hemicrania. Attacks are much shorter than in cluster headache, lasting for only seconds or minutes. Paroxysmal hemicrania does not respond to cluster headache treatments. However, it does respond – almost magically – to an anti-inflammatory drug called indometacin.

Causes of cluster headache

Despite current research, we do not yet know the cause and mechanisms of cluster headache. The timing of cluster headache attacks is a fascinating phenomenon. The striking annual regularity with the changes of seasons and attacks at exact times each day during a bout suggest links with circadian rhythms or the body clock. Research has focused on this biological clock, which is controlled by a part of the brain called the hypothalamus. Recently, positron emission tomography (an imaging technique, also known as PET) has suggested that this area is abnormally active during attacks of cluster headache and may generate the pain.

Cluster headache may be inherited in about five per cent of cases. We are not sure how significant a genetic link is in relation to other factors such as environmental triggers.

Triggers for cluster headache

Triggers are mostly significant in chronic cluster headache or during a bout of episodic cluster headache. They do not tend to provoke new bouts. Here are the main ones.

- *Alcohol* can trigger an attack within half an hour in about 90 per cent of those with cluster headache. This is quite different from migraine, in which the effect is delayed. Alcohol is not usually a problem when you are outside a cluster bout. Some people recognize when they are emerging from a cluster episode by their tolerance to alcohol. Specific foods don't appear to trigger cluster headaches.
- *Smoking* is associated with cluster headache. Sixty per cent of people with cluster headache are smokers, and a further 20 per cent have smoked previously. Despite this association, smoking does not cause cluster headache or trigger individual attacks. Stopping smoking is not guaranteed to help but it is highly recommended for general health. There is some suggestion that heavy smokers are more likely to develop chronic cluster headache.
- *Sleep* is a definite trigger, with up to three quarters of attacks occurring at night. They often coincide with REM (rapid eye movement) sleep only an hour or two after falling asleep. You may dread the night because attacks often wake you. There may be an association with sleep apnoea, which is when breathing stops for short periods during sleep.
- *Elevated temperature*, either due to environmental temperature changes or to exercising, can provoke attacks.

- *Exposure to volatile substances* such as solvents, oil-based paints and other chemicals with strong smells can act as a trigger. Nitroglycerine, histamines and monosodium glutamate are also triggers.
- *Relaxation* can provoke attacks. Unlike migraine, stress is not a trigger with cluster headaches, which often start when you relax or go to sleep.
- *Air travel* is another potential trigger, possibly related to changes in altitude or changes in time zones, which upset the biological clock.
- *Head injury* one or two weeks before the first cluster headache occurs in about one to two per cent. It is not regarded as a typical trigger and is difficult to assess, because head injury is common in the general population.

Does cluster headache improve?

Your pattern of cluster headache is impossible to predict. Some people have recurring attacks of pain, whereas others enjoy remissions for a decade or more. We don't know why episodic cluster headache evolves to the chronic form in a minority – about ten per cent. Fortunately, the general pattern for all cluster headache types is one of improvement over the course of a life time. Encouragingly, attacks can become much less frequent as you get older and often disappear altogether.

9

Coping with cluster headache

Cluster headache is an excruciating headache. It is called 'suicide headache', and with good reason. Unfortunately, self-help treatments don't work. Over-the-counter painkillers and tablets are not absorbed via the stomach quickly enough to provide relief. You can try a self-help and non-drug approach, because anything that promotes general health and well being may help you. However, we have no scientific evidence of specific benefits.

You need medical help to cope with cluster headache, and a visit to your doctor is important for diagnosis. It is best if your doctor understands your condition so that you can work together to find effective treatments. General practitioners (GPs) are supportive, but few will have encountered cluster headache in general practice. If cluster headache is not recognized it can be mistreated as migraine. Do seek another opinion and referral to a headache specialist doctor if you need more help. Although there is no cure, medical treatments can help enormously.

Coping with cluster headache with medical treatments

Doctors use treatments in two ways. Symptomatic (acute) treatments deal with cluster headache once it starts and preventatives are taken daily. The two types of treatment are used together to achieve maximum benefit. Preventatives are continued for at least two weeks after a cluster bout, to be confident that it has completely finished. Sometimes specialists use a short course of preventatives such as steroids to abort the cluster headaches quickly. Afterward a maintenance therapy may be used until the end of the cluster bout, or continuously in the case of chronic cluster headache.

Treatments for cluster headache symptoms

Generally, tablet forms of medications are not effective because they don't work quickly enough.

Sumatriptan injection

Trials show that sumatriptan injection is effective in about 75 per cent of people with cluster headache. It can stop cluster attacks in 15–30 minutes. Sumatriptan injection is licensed for use in cluster headache and is available on prescription. Although many people don't like injecting themselves, the auto-injector device is simple to use. Generally, the discomfort is minimal compared with the pain of the headache.

The injection can only be used twice in 24 hours, with at least two hours between doses, which is why it is combined with other treatments. It can be used long term in chronic cluster headache. Sumatriptan can't be used by people with heart problems or high blood pressure. Medication over-use headache can occur in the treatment of cluster headache and is more likely if you or your family have migraine.

Susan, 34

'The injections work well for me and the attack has usually gone in 15 minutes. I can feel it beginning to work before then, which is such a relief. I always carry the injection with me in case of an attack so I can use it at the start. It doesn't work as well otherwise. I use a lot of injections when I'm in a cluster. The last bout was the first one in three years and I only ever use the injections during cluster bouts. The injections are expensive, but my GP is very supportive, as he knows how devastating my cluster headaches are without them.'

Oxygen therapy

Oxygen delivered at 100 per cent with a high flow rate can stop cluster attacks within 15–30 minutes. It is not specifically licensed for use in cluster headache, being more commonly used at low flow rates for chest or breathing problems. However, recent research suggests that oxygen should be widely available for cluster headache. It can help more than two thirds of people and is safe to use without any side effects. Once your diagnosis is confirmed, your doctor can prescribe it 'off-label'. Oxygen is easy to use but it is vital to obtain the correct equipment and use it properly if you are to gain benefit.

Tips for obtaining and using oxygen therapy

- Your doctor can send a Home Oxygen Order Form (HOOF) to your regional supplier. If an initial form is completed as an emergency order, the oxygen should be delivered to your home on the same day. The doctor can complete a second non-urgent request at the same time, to ensure ongoing supply.
- Make sure you are using oxygen at a high enough rate. You need 100 per cent oxygen at seven to 12 litres per minute with a non-rebreathe mask. Experiment to find the effective rate. Adjust the head strap for a snug fit. Masks with holes are not effective.
- Sit upright and lean slightly forward, if possible. Follow the safety instructions and remember not to smoke near the cylinder.
- Try to use oxygen early in an attack. This gives the treatment the best chance of working. It can work quickly within five to ten minutes, but you may need to experiment. People often use it for about 15–20 minutes. Keep using the oxygen until the attack has gone completely – otherwise it can come back.
- If you find oxygen to be effective, ask your doctor for a standard oxygen cylinder for home use and a portable one for elsewhere. Both types come with built in regulators so that you can obtain the high flow rate.
- An oxygen cylinder may not last long if your attacks are frequent, so ask your doctor for a second cylinder. Always have the empty cylinder replaced promptly, so that you are not caught without a supply.
- Oxygen concentrator machines that provide one to five litres per minute are insufficient and ineffective for treatment of cluster headache.

Daniel, 31
'Oxygen was a great discovery. I didn't think it worked at first, but then I realized I was not using the right mask and the flow rate was too low. My GP got that changed, and I now have a cylinder in my office and at home next to my bed. I am never far from one if an attack comes on. I can feel it working within a few minutes and I usually continue the oxygen for about 15 minutes until the attack goes completely. It is helpful at night and means I can get some sleep instead of getting exhausted with the pain.'

Other acute treatments

Sumatriptan or zolmitriptan nasal sprays can work well although not usually as quickly as oxygen and sumatriptan injection. Other drugs sometimes used are octreotide by subcutaneous injection and lidocaine in nose drops or a spray. In terms of self-help techniques during an attack, most people are too agitated to think about relaxation or deep breathing exercises. No complementary therapies have been shown to be an effective alternative to medication. Application of hot or cold packs and biofeedback may help to reduce the pain in addition to standard treatments.

Preventative treatments for cluster headache

Currently, the most effective preventatives are verapamil, methysergide and steroids, all given in tablet formulation with specially tailored dose plans.

Verapamil

The first choice is often verapamil. This is used in low doses to treat high blood pressure and heart conditions, including angina, but it is also effective at preventing cluster headache. Do not be alarmed that high doses may be required to control your cluster headache. The doses start low and are gradually increased as necessary. The effective dose is maintained for the anticipated duration of the cluster and then gradually reduced over one to two weeks. It can be increased if attacks recur and may be used long term in chronic cluster attacks. We don't have any evidence that long-term use in episodic cluster headache can stop further bouts.

At high doses verapamil can affect the heart in some people. So heart tracings called ECGs (electrocardiograms) are done regularly to monitor any changes. Other side effects include constipation and gum problems, and so a high-fibre diet and good dental hygiene are important.

Methysergide

Methysergide is specifically licensed for prevention of cluster headache and migraine. It is very effective, particularly for short-bout cluster headaches. It is used under close supervision by specialist doctors in gradually increasing doses, if tolerated. It must not be used for more than six months without a one-month 'drug holiday', because long-term use may cause damage to major organs such as heart, lungs and kidneys. Short-term side effects of leg cramps, abdominal discomfort and nausea usually stop with gradual dose increase and continued use.

Steroids

A five-day course of prednisolone in reducing doses is effective at rapidly stopping cluster attacks. This short-term prevention can be helpful while waiting for other longer term treatments (e.g. verapamil or methysergide) to take effect. Unfortunately, headaches usually recur when treatment is stopped, and the long-term side effects of possible infection and bone loss limit ongoing steroid use. Short-term side effects such as gastric irritation can be lessened by using a special tablet formulation called 'enteric coated'.

Other preventative treatments

Other preventative treatments include lithium, which can be moderately effective. Blood levels needs monitoring to ensure that levels of the drug are adequate and to avoid toxic effects.

A half or a whole ergotamine suppository was a standard cluster headache treatment for many years, used for short bouts of cluster headache. Taken at bedtime, ergotamine may stop some night-time attacks. There is little evidence from clinical practice or research to suggest that pizotifen, sodium valproate, gabapentin, melatonin and botulinum toxin are effective treatments for cluster headache prevention.

Small-scale studies of a nasal spray form of capsaicin called civamide suggest moderate benefit. There is interest in studying topiramate, an anti-epileptic that is helpful in preventing migraine. Some people have experienced benefit from greater occipital nerve injections of steroids or anaesthetic.

Surgical treatments for cluster headaches

Surgical treatments are considered only for those with frequent cluster attacks (usually the chronic form) when standard medical treatments don't work. There is no guarantee of benefit and all surgery can have risks. We need much more research in this area and so far only small numbers of people have been treated.

Continuous stimulation of the occipital nerve at the back of the head, via an electrode placed under the scalp, can be of benefit in reducing painful attacks. Because the hypothalamus has been shown in brain scans to be a possible origin of cluster headache, there is also current interest in stimulating this area directly. This is called 'deep brain stimulation' and has shown some success in a small number of people with chronic cluster headache.

James, 44

'My cluster attacks always start with slight "niggles" before a full-blown cluster begins. This is now the signal for me to start verapamil. I have used it for two previous bouts and it really helped. I still had some attacks in the early weeks, but somehow they didn't take hold. I was able to start reducing the verapamil after six weeks and they didn't start up again. Previous bouts tended to last 12 weeks, so this was a great improvement.'

Tips for coping with cluster headaches

- Get medical help and referral to a headache specialist. It is important that you find and work with a supportive doctor.
- A diagnosis of cluster headache can feel devastating and you may feel isolated. You are not alone and help is available.
- Get in touch with the Organization for the Understanding of Cluster Headache (OUCH). This excellent charity provides useful information about coping with cluster headache. (See Useful addresses at the end of this book.)
- Report any side effects and changes in health to your doctor. Some treatments used for cluster headache need to be monitored.
- Keep a diary of headaches and associated symptoms. Diaries are helpful to assess whether the treatments are working.
- Use symptomatic treatments as early on in an attack as possible. Be prepared with your treatment for the next attack.
- Begin preventatives early in a cluster bout. They are more likely to prevent headaches quickly and may help symptomatic treatments to work better.
- If you sense that a bout of cluster headache is about to start, see your doctor to obtain your prescriptions and oxygen supply.
- Identify triggers if possible and avoid them if you can (e.g. alcohol). You don't need to stop exercising unless this is a trigger for you. If getting over-heated is a trigger, then take care to keep the central heating turned down low and take cool rather than hot baths and showers.
- Don't take naps during the day if you get night time attacks. Naps may trigger daytime attacks too.
- Give up smoking. Although this may not affect the pattern of

cluster headache, it reduces chances of other illnesses such as heart disease and you may not have to stop other treatments in the future.

- During a cluster bout, make allowances for how you feel. Don't plan activities that you don't need to do.
- Tell friends and colleagues about your cluster headache. During a bout you may just be concentrating on getting through the pain – those close to you will not understand what you are experiencing. Colleagues are more likely to be supportive (especially if you miss time from work) if you have explained what is happening.
- Let others know if there is anything that they can do to help. Your loved ones will be horrified at what you endure. Your colleagues will be scared of what they may have to witness. Everyone will feel terrible that there is little they can do. If there is something they can do – perhaps getting the hot and cold packs – then tell them. If it is best for them to simply stay away, then gently explain that too.

10

Daily headaches

Pauline, 42
Pauline rang me to volunteer for a clinical study on menstrual migraine. She had severe migraine at period time and less severe weekly attacks that she treated with triptans. I asked her about any other headaches. She told me that she also got fuzzy headaches every day and took painkillers for them most days. All her headaches were really getting her down.

Daily or nearly daily headache affects about four per cent of the adult population, mainly women. More than three quarters have had episodic headaches previously. Few people seek help from their doctor, and by the time they do they may have endured pain for a long time.

Reasons for developing daily headaches

Daily headache is a label (not a diagnosis) for headache of any type that regularly occurs on more than 15 days each month. We don't know why some people develop daily headaches and others escape, but several factors contribute.

Over-use of painkillers or triptans

Over-use of these medications can lead to medication over-use headache if you are regularly treating yourself on two or three days each week.

Changes in other headache

Changes in other headache such as migraine, tension-type headache and cluster headache from episodic to chronic forms can result in daily headaches. Development of additional headaches can be due to over-use of drugs. This often occurs in so-called 'chronic migraine', when migraine-like headache and symptoms occur on more than 15 days each month.

Underlying trauma, diseases and infections

These include sinusitis, neck and jaw problems, and temporal arteritis (a form of inflammation of arteries that is more common in older people). Frequent unchanged headaches for many years make a brain tumour unlikely. If headaches become progressively worse or are accompanied by other symptoms, see your doctor.

Rare daily headaches

These can be caused by high or low pressure in the brain. Other rare headaches (e.g. hemicrania continua) and new persistent daily headache can be of sudden onset. These are best assessed and treated by a specialist.

The influence of other risk factors

A combination of risk factors can influence any of the other reasons, and these include:

- poor sleep, including snoring and other sleep disturbances;
- caffeine intake;
- obesity;
- genetic factors;
- thyroid problems;
- anxiety and depression;
- stressful life events; and
- being divorced, separated or widowed.

Other unknown reasons

Not everyone who has daily headaches will be over-using medications or have an identifiable cause for their headache. Other biological and psychological mechanisms that we do not yet understand may be the reason.

Coping with daily headaches

If your headaches are most days you are not alone. Here are the key aims as you cope with your headache.

Get help from a headache specialist

Do not put off seeking help. Daily headaches are more difficult to treat the longer you have had them. Sometimes, experts find it hard to distinguish headache types, especially if medication over-use is present.

However, you can get help to prevent some headaches and to treat properly those you cannot avoid.

Identify your headache

You may have more than one type of headache. Keep a diary. Migraine, tension-type headaches and medication over-use headaches can all co-exist. If headaches can be identified and tackled separately, then it may be that by improving one type of headache the other(s) will benefit too.

Treat non-migraine headaches first

Tension-type headache and medication over-use headache typically make migraine worse and less likely to respond to any management strategies. The result is different types of headaches on most days and a tendency to over-use medication.

Deal with other medical issues

Any uncontrolled problem is likely to worsen headache. Consider all your health issues and tackle them separately, but remember that they affect you as a whole person.

Identify and avoid over-use of symptomatic treatments

Medication over-use is discussed in Chapters 11 and 12.

Identify and avoid other risk factors

This is not always possible but maintaining a healthy weight, getting enough sleep and cutting down on caffeine intake may help.

Find different ways of coping with the pain

You may need specialist help from a pain centre or clinic to deal with chronic pain. Combinations of physical and psychological approaches may be used to help, and your doctor may refer you. (See Chapter 20.)

11

Medication over-use headache

Penny, 35
'I have headaches all the time and I almost rattle with the amount of pills that I am taking. They don't really help, but if I don't take them every day then the headache is worse.'

Painkillers and triptans are part of our weaponry in the war against headaches and migraine. They are important to help us cope. However, use must be limited and appropriate, otherwise – instead of helping – the treatment makes the problem worse. This is called 'medication over-use headache' (MOH).

What is medication over-use headache?

Symptomatic medications taken on two or three days each week on average, over several months, can cause MOH. Medications prescribed and taken daily to *prevent* headaches and migraine are not the problem. The issue is with medications used to *treat symptoms* of headache when it occurs. *All* symptomatic treatment may cause MOH. These include:

- opioids (e.g. codeine and dihydrocodeine),
- combination painkillers (paracetamol with codeine or aspirin combined with caffeine),
- ergotamine,
- triptans used for migraine (e.g. almotriptan, eletriptan, naratriptan, rizatriptan, sumatriptan, zolmitriptan and frovatriptan),
- non-steroidal anti-inflammatory drugs (e.g. aspirin, ibuprofen, naproxen and diclofenac) and
- paracetamol.

Amount of medication needed to cause medication over-use headache

Low doses of symptomatic treatments on frequent days causes greater risk of MOH than large doses infrequently. The number of days of dosing in a month are important – not the number of doses in a day.

This means that you can treat severe headache confidently using maximum daily doses of medication if necessary, but not too often. The guidance is as follows.

- Triptans, opioids such as codeine, combination painkillers and ergotamine should not be taken on ten or more days per month.
- Simple painkillers such as aspirin, paracetamol and ibuprofen should not be taken on 15 or more days per month.

Features of medication over-use headache

Studies suggest 65 per cent of people with MOH have migraine, 27 per cent have tension-type headache and the rest have both or other headaches. The MOH may be similar to your usual headache and/or it may be an oppressive dull ache that is constant or may wax and wane.

MOH is not progressive. It occurs most days and is often worse in the morning when medication levels in the blood are lowest. It can be aggravated by mental or physical effort such as exercise. Medication for symptoms or prevention and other treatments have little effect on it. If you try to stop medications your headache gets much worse.

Other symptoms may include tiredness, lethargy, irritability, forgetfulness, difficulty sleeping and constipation. Nausea and vomiting are less of a problem. Your daily activities may or may not be badly affected.

Who gets medication over-use headache?

Studies show MOH affects about two per cent of the general population. It affects five times as many women than men and also may occur in children and teenagers. It is frequent, increasing and happens worldwide, although the medications used vary.

MOH is common in those who seek help for their headaches. It is reported in at least ten per cent of those attending headache centres in Europe and up to 70 per cent in the USA. People often say that they have tried every medication and nothing works. They may have been to many doctors or therapists and none was able to help. Frequently, they are depressed about their headaches.

MOH develops in headache-prone people. People who do not have tension-type headaches or migraine do not tend to develop MOH if they use painkillers for other conditions such as arthritis or back pain. People with these conditions who also have migraine should take particular care. MOH is less common with cluster headache, but may occur in those who have migraine or a family history of migraine.

Mechanisms of medication over-use headache

Addiction, a craving or a physical dependence is not usual with simple painkillers or triptans. It can happen with codeine and other opioids, caffeine, ergotamine, dihydroergotamine, barbiturates and sedatives. Psychological factors are important because you expect pain relief by taking medication, and this can be a hard habit to break. This can even be learned in childhood if your parents readily took painkillers.

The predisposition to MOH in those with migraine and tension-type headaches could be genetic or due to biological changes in the brain. Specific mechanisms are unknown and may vary. Regular and repeated exposure to a drug could affect biochemical or nerve function and change pain receptor activation in the brain. Pain receptors may become switched on to give you a permanent sensation of headache pain or they could have a low threshold to produce pain.

Tips for preventing medication over-use headache

Medication over-use is often overlooked. You may be treating headaches with over-the-counter medications and doctors may not warn you in advance of prescribing drugs. Prevention while a headache is intermittent is best. Here are tips to help you.

- Limit triptan use for migraine to a maximum of ten days per month.
- Limit painkillers to a maximum of 15 days per month.
- Remember that it is the number of days that you treat that is important – not the number of doses in a day.
- Avoid any drugs containing caffeine, codeine or other combination painkillers.
- Avoid barbiturates and tranquillizers.
- Avoid changing one drug for another. This is just as risky for developing MOH.
- Treat migraine early and with high enough doses of medication. Add in anti-sickness medications to help nausea and – importantly – to prevent your gut from shutting down.
- If your usual medication is not very effective or becomes less so, then check that you are using it correctly (i.e. at the right time,

the right route and the right dose). Change your treatments if necessary.

- Keep a diary. Record all headaches and *all* medications you take, even on days that you do not have a headache. A bad month or two can happen from time to time – the concern is month after month of frequent headaches and frequent treatments.

- Distinguish migraine from other headaches. You may be treating headaches that would otherwise have gone away and therefore taking more treatments than you need to.

- Don't take treatments for headaches just in case one might develop. People often do this. It does not work and can increase your risk of MOH. It is much better to take a step back and assess your triggers, ensure that you have treatments that work if a headache develops and use preventatives if necessary.

- Be aware of the potential for MOH to develop quickly – even over weeks in some people.

- Don't delay seeking help if you think you need it. The longer that MOH continues, the more difficult it is to treat.

- Be honest with your doctor about the amount of medication you are using. Repeat prescription and purchases over-the-counter must all be discussed.

- Start preventatives and other strategies when headaches are becoming frequent but before you start over-using your medications. Preventatives are more likely to work and may reduce your risk of developing MOH.

- You could be at higher risk of MOH if you have other medical conditions. Get proper treatment if necessary. Be especially careful if you have to take painkillers for other conditions, which will often be made worse by MOH.

12

Treating medication over-use headache

If you have medication over-use headache (MOH), continued over-use of medications to treat symptoms will make your headaches worse and not better. Preventative medications and any complementary strategies you try are unlikely to be very successful. The only way to change this is to break the cycle and to stop the medications.

If you can do this then there is a very good chance of significant improvement. Studies show that in the first six months around 70 per cent of people will have at least half the number of headache days. Many have even fewer. So it is really worth aiming for.

Tackling your MOH does not mean that you can't use medications for headache symptoms again, but in the short term you must stop. Most people find when their headaches become less frequent, medications – if used carefully and cautiously – become effective again.

How to stop medications

Stopping medications completely may be the best and quickest way for triptans, ergotamine and painkillers that do not contain codeine.

Talk to your doctor if you are using codeine-containing medications or other types of drugs. A gradual withdrawal programme may be recommended, depending on the amount of codeine and type of drug you are over-using. You could start by taking your medication daily at fixed times only and then reduce the amount gradually over several weeks.

Drug withdrawal can usually be done as an outpatient with the support of your doctor and family. Referral to a specialist may be helpful, and sometimes hospitalization is advised to give you extra support over the first week, depending on what drugs you have been using. Drinking lots of water is particularly important.

What to expect when you stop medications

Because your body has become used to regular medications, you are likely to experience some 'withdrawal' symptoms when you stop the drugs. These include:

- aggravation of your headache, which temporarily can be severe;
- nausea and vomiting within a couple of days, which should gradually improve; and
- anxiety, restlessness, nervousness, insomnia and/or racing pulse.

Some people may worry about having fits and hallucinations when they withdraw from triptans and over-the-counter painkillers; fortunately, this is not reported.

At their worst, severe symptoms last an average of four days. They usually start within two days of stopping the medication and begin to improve within seven to ten days for triptan over-use, two to three weeks for painkiller over-use, and two to four weeks with opioids such as codeine. If you have been using combination painkillers or mixing painkillers with triptans, then the whole withdrawal process can take six to 12 weeks. You should start to feel better during this time though, especially when the daily headaches begin to lift.

Supportive medical strategies

All painkillers and triptans must be stopped completely – otherwise supportive strategies will not help. Research doesn't indicate which are best strategies, and they may vary between specialists.

- Naproxen can be used to aid recovery from MOH and replace your usual method of pain control. This non-steroidal anti-inflammatory drug is prescribed in a six-week reducing regimen. It is taken daily at fixed times with food. If it irritates your stomach, then your doctor can prescribe additional medication.
- Amitriptyline can help to ease pain. It is prescribed over three months, starting with a low dose at night and increasing gradually.
- Anti-sickness medications such as metoclopramide and domperidone can be helpful. They can be taken as suppositories if necessary.
- Migraine preventatives, including beta-blockers such as propanolol or topiramate, may be used. We need further studies to assess the best time to consider these. Some specialists commence before medication withdrawal whereas others wait.
- Steroids such as prednisolone may be used in a reducing dose over six days.

- Greater occipital nerve injections of lidocaine and steroids may provide some relief of headache severity over two weeks to cover the worst period of withdrawal.
- Triptans may be prescribed by your doctor to treat severe migraine attacks soon after withdrawal, providing it was *not* triptans that you were over-using.

Dealing with headaches in the future

Headaches that remain after withdrawal are usually more obvious. A properly diagnosed headache and not a fuzzy, daily MOH is more likely to respond to medications, if they are used properly. Preventative treatments may be started and, although they have failed in the past, they may now be successful.

Ongoing, regular follow up with your doctor and maintaining a diary is recommended, because your recovery will continue for some months. Studies show a relapse rate of up to 40 per cent within five years, so you must be on your guard. This is most likely during the first year, especially if you had a mixture of migraine and other headaches and/or combined your medications. We need more studies to find out why some people relapse and others don't.

If you are not taking medications and your headache didn't improve after withdrawal, your doctor may refer you to a headache specialist to confirm the diagnosis.

Coping with medication withdrawal

Stopping medication is never easy but it will be worth it. You won't get a 'miracle cure', but hopefully you can return to less frequent headaches, which respond to treatment. The daily headache should disappear and you can look forward to headache-free days.

It seems unfair that you must prepare for even worse headaches during drug withdrawal. Remember, though, that it will only be for a relatively short time. Compared with the months and perhaps years that you may have battled with your headaches, the worst will be over quickly.

An awareness of what to expect can increase your ability to cope with withdrawal. The withdrawal may disrupt your life temporarily, so – apart from your willpower – gather whatever support you need to help you.

The tips provided in the information box should increase your chances of success. Good luck!

Tips for coping with medication withdrawal

- Choose a time to suit you, so that you have the best chance of success and can ensure that support is in place. Also, try to choose a time of low stress if you can, but especially not when you are about to move house or have a big change at work. You might need some annual leave.
- If you are finding reasons not to do this, then deal with those reasons first. There may never be a perfect time!
- Plan to stop *all* painkillers or triptans *completely* unless you are on a medication-reducing schedule from your doctor. If the medication withdrawal is not complete, then you are more likely to relapse.
- Do as little as possible *or* keep busy. *Definitely* pamper yourself. There is no right or wrong way. Everyone is different. It will depend on how you feel.
- Ask for help if you need it, for example help with childcare.
- Tell your family and friends. You will need their support and encouragement. Also inform colleagues at work.
- Discuss your medication withdrawal with your doctor. You will need support and perhaps some prescriptions, so plan a regular review. If you do not have a supportive doctor, seek a different one. Also consider going to a specialist headache centre.
- Find non-drug strategies to cope that are not painkillers. Some people find acupuncture, counselling or the principles of cognitive behavioural therapy helpful. Start relaxation and stress management therapies early on in the process. This will put you in a stronger position for coping in the long term.
- Keep a diary, even if it makes horrid reading. Even daily headache changes from day to day. After the medication withdrawal you will see how far you have come. It is always encouraging to see headache-free days, patterns become more obvious and it is easier to target treatment.
- Don't be ashamed. It is better to be open and honest about what is happening – both with yourself and those who are trying to help you.
- If frequent headaches don't go or they disappear and return again, have a chat with your doctor.
- Be positive and believe that you can do it. Even if you don't succeed you will be in a better position for success next time, because you will know what to expect and how medication withdrawal affects you.

13

Headaches, hormones and periods

About 80 per cent of people attending the City of London Migraine Clinic are women. This is because of the influence of women's hormones on migraine. Oestrogen and progesterone rise and fall to create menstrual cycles during your reproductive life. At the menopause, when periods stop, these fluctuations dwindle. If you are sensitive to these normal changes you can get headaches and migraine. There does not have to be anything wrong with either you or your hormones! This chapter looks at hormones and headaches in relation to menstrual migraine, premenstrual syndrome and contraception.

Women, hormones and headaches

There is plenty of evidence suggesting female sex hormones have a lot to answer for. Perhaps you recognize yourself in the following.

- Until puberty boys and girls are equally affected by migraine. After puberty, when hormones change, more girls are affected.
- Migraine is three times more common in women during their reproductive years. It affects up to a quarter of women and only around eight per cent of men. It peaks in women in their forties when their hormones are changing.
- Fifty per cent of women with migraine notice a link with their periods.
- Many women notice headaches and migraine during the pill-free week when they are on the oral contraceptive pill.
- Around two thirds of women find that migraine improves during pregnancy.
- Migraine usually stops or improves after the menopause.
- Hormone replacement therapy can either help migraine or make it worse.

The burden of coping is difficult for women if headache patterns alter as hormones fluctuate. These fluctuations can be caused by your own hormone cycles or by external hormones you take for contraception or hormone replacement therapy. However, hormones are unlikely to be the sole headache trigger, so it is important to keep a perspective and not to forget non-hormonal triggers and lifestyle management, and to avoid medication over-use.

Menstrual migraine

This is migraine without aura at period time. Attacks start either one or two days before bleeding or on the first, second or third day. The attacks occur in at least two out of three menstrual cycles on average. Menstrual migraine is only properly diagnosed with diary records kept for at least three cycles. These are also essential for assessing response to treatments and the best timing for them.

Types of menstrual migraine

There are two subtypes.

- In pure menstrual migraine, attacks occur exclusively around the first day of the period and at *no other time* during the cycle. It is rare and affects less than ten per cent of women who have migraine.
- In menstrually related migraine, attacks occur around the first day of the period and *additionally* at other times during the cycle. This type affects up to 40 per cent of women who have migraine.

Women attending headache clinics often report that menstrual attacks are more severe than non-menstrual ones. Associated with more disability, nausea and vomiting, they are often less responsive to treatments, last longer and recur over several days.

Causes of menstrual migraine

The causes of menstrual migraine are unknown. Migraine triggers including environment, genetic tendency and changes in brain chemicals may combine with the additional trigger of hormone changes. There is no evidence of abnormal changes or levels in your hormones, which is why doctors do not do blood tests. You are just likely to be more sensitive to the normal hormonal changes.

There are two main hormones produced by the ovaries: oestrogen and progesterone. Studies in the 1970s suggested changes in oestrogen are most important for migraine. More recent work supports the 'oestrogen withdrawal' theory for some but not all women. This is the gradual drop in oestrogen that naturally occurs before a period. Oestrogen is unlikely to be the only factor, and the release of other chemicals called prostaglandins can also be associated with painful, heavy periods and menstrual migraines.

Treating menstrual migraine symptoms

There are no medications specifically for treating the symptoms of menstrual migraine. Clinical studies show that all of the anti-migraine drugs (triptans) can help with menstrual migraine. Some women find that standard painkillers and anti-sickness medications will suffice. Make sure that you are using your treatments optimally.

Preventing menstrual migraine with non-hormonal strategies

Menstrual migraine attacks are stubborn – you may eliminate most migraine attacks to find that the menstrual one still remains. There are no specifically licensed preventatives and research evidence is limited. Here are the main approaches used, and they may need to be combined.

- Non-drug approaches, including lifestyle management and trigger avoidance, are important. Menstruation is another step on the trigger ladder that can tip you over the migraine threshold. (The migraine threshold is discussed in Chapter 4.)
- Standard preventative treatments such as amitriptyline or propanolol may be helpful for both menstrual and non-menstrual attacks.
- Non-steroidal anti-inflammatory drugs (e.g. mefenamic acid), started two days before the period and continued throughout (or on the days of heavy flow), can help by stopping release of prostaglandins. Naproxen is an alternative, but it does not help with heavy bleeding.
- Preventative triptans have been used in research trials with some benefit. Specialists may recommend short courses, but additional triptans should not be used simultaneously.
- Magnesium daily can be effective but diarrhoea may be a side effect.

Preventing menstrual migraine with hormonal strategies

Severe menstrual migraine does not necessarily mean that hormonal treatment is required. Whether hormonal treatment is the best option for you depends on your individual circumstances, including need for contraception, other medical conditions (e.g. depression or high blood pressure) and how well your symptomatic treatments work. Hormonal treatments may work better if non-hormonal triggers are eliminated, but we do not have scientific evidence for this.

Hormonal strategies that may be considered are as follows.

- Combined hormonal contraceptives, used by 'tricycling' or continuous pill dosing (see the section entitled 'Effect of hormonal

contraception on headaches and migraine', p. 76), may be options if
you do not have migraine with aura at other times in your menstrual
cycle.

- Progestogen-only contraceptives such as depot medroxyproges-
terone acetate injections and the newer Cerazette® pill, which stop
ovulation, may be useful. Periods are likely to stop and the oestrogen withdrawal trigger is lessened. This does not happen with the
implants or the older pills, with which the rise and fall of oestrogen
during the cycle continues.

- The Mirena® intra-uterine system is helpful in some women. It
reduces the heavy period trigger by making the womb lining
thinner. After some spot bleeding with early use, periods usually
become lighter and may stop. The prostaglandin trigger for migraine
is also reduced.

- Oestrogen supplements may stop the oestrogen withdrawal trigger.
Supplements are not hormonal replacement therapy, in which
additional progestogens are required to protect your womb from
oestrogen. Your doctor or specialist may prescribe supplements 'off-
label' as gel or skin patches to be used around your period. You can
only use this strategy if there are no contraindications for your use
of oestrogen, you have predictable periods and you are ovulating
regularly. This can be checked by blood tests. A home use fertility
monitor may be helpful to check ovulation and predict optimal
timing of treatment.

Preventing menstrual migraine with surgery

Surgery might seem the obvious solution to menstrual migraine.
Unfortunately, it is not that simple, and hysterectomy is not recommended for migraine alone.

Limited data suggest that hysterectomy with or without removal of
the ovaries can actually aggravate migraine. In one study two thirds
of women found that migraine worsened. This is because hormone
cycles are controlled by a part of the brain called the hypothalamus.
Hysterectomy removes only the end organs, or the last part of the
process, and it does not tackle the root of the problem in the brain.

If you need a hysterectomy for other medical reasons (e.g.
fibroids – growths in the womb), hormone replacement therapy may
be recommended. There are some formulations of hormone replacement therapy that are less likely to aggravate your migraine attacks.
(See Chapter 15.)

Denise, 44

Denise – a secretary and single mother of two – had been having migraine without aura since around the age of 12, when her periods began. Her daughter had started having headaches, and Denise was hoping that they would not follow her own pattern of severe migraines with her periods. Denise's mother also had migraine, which improved when her periods stopped at the menopause. Denise used to feel that this could come soon enough for her and had been wondering whether she should just get everything over with and have a hysterectomy.

Migraine was always worse for Denise at stressful times such as starting a new job and the terrible time when she got divorced. She remembers excruciating migraines during the pill-free week when she was using the oral contraceptive pill, but in contrast she was migraine-free during both pregnancies. Denise always noticed a link with migraine and her periods, and this has become worse in recent years. Her periods, still regular, had become heavier and more painful. Migraine attacks were usually much more painful during her periods, lasted up to three days, and were often associated with vomiting. She had to go to bed and miss work. Grandparents and neighbours were called at short notice to look after the children, making her feel guilty, which only makes things worse. Her general practitioner (GP), who diagnosed migraine, pre-scribed a triptan – a specific anti-migraine medication. Denise came to see us the City of London Migraine Clinic when the medication stopped working and she lived in dread of her period each month.

The specialist confirmed the diagnosis of migraine and reassured Denise that there were various strategies worth trying. The doctor advised that hormone tests, brain scans or operations would not help, and asked her to keep a diary for three months. In the meantime, Denise was encouraged to be strict about non-hormonal trigger factors and lifestyle issues. At her follow-up appointment, her diaries confirmed menstrually related migraine. Although non-menstrual attacks were greatly reduced and better controlled using aspirin and domperidone (an anti-sickness drug), menstrual attacks always needed a triptan repeated over several days. The doctor suggested increasing the dose of the triptan combined with domperidone and using them earlier in the attack. Mefenamic acid (a non-steroidal anti-inflammatory drug) was added for a few days only around period time to help both the migraine and also the heavier, painful periods.

These strategies, combined with Denise's efforts at managing non-hormonal triggers such as missed meals, overtiredness, dehydration and stress meant that she has regained control of her migraines and her life. She no longer lives in dread of her next period. If migraine occurs, her medication usually works well and she no longer misses time from work.

Premenstrual syndrome

Premenstrual syndrome (PMS) describes a range of symptoms in the week or so before your period, which usually subside when it starts. They often include tension-type headache and migraines. PMS is common and affects around two thirds of menstruating women. Although you might think that you are imagining things, this is a recognized syndrome. Symptoms include:

- tiredness,
- difficulty sleeping,
- irritability,
- being tearful,
- depression,
- poor concentration,
- breast tenderness,
- abdominal bloating,
- appetite change,
- muscle and joint pain and
- acne.

Headaches and premenstrual syndrome

Headaches and migraines may be linked to the other PMS symptoms but we are not sure how. Migraine does not necessarily have the regularity and specific timing of menstrual migraine and the mechanisms may be different. We do not know whether specific changes in the hormone cycles cause PMS symptoms in some women. There are no hormone tests to diagnosis PMS, because the fluctuations are part of the normal menstrual cycle.

Coping with headaches and premenstrual syndrome

Some evidence suggests that the worse the PMS, the worse the headaches. So if you can reduce your PMS symptoms, your headaches may also improve. Diet and self-help measures may help both. The following measures may particularly help with PMS.

- Reduce salt and sugar in your diet.
- Take multivitamins and supplements such as vitamin B complex, calcium and magnesium.

- Take herbal supplements such as evening primrose oil and *Agnus castus*.

If you need medical help to deal with PMS symptoms, then your doctor may suggest one of the contraceptive pills that stop ovulation. In some women this can lessen the symptoms.

Headaches and contraception

There are three groups of contraceptives: combined hormonal, progestogen-only and non-hormonal.

Combined hormonal contraception

Combined hormonal contraceptives (CHCs) include pills, patches and vaginal rings that contain both oestrogen and progestogen. They are safe and effective for the majority of women, even those with migraine. However, studies of combined oral contraceptive pills show an increased risk of ischaemic stroke (in which the brain is deprived of its blood supply) in young women. The risk increases with higher dose oestrogen preparations. Overall, the chances of getting a stroke are low. An annual estimate is up to four per 100,000 healthy women who do not smoke. This is doubled to around eight if women are using combined oral contraceptive pills.

Studies have shown that migraine *with* aura (but not migraine *without* aura) is a marker for an individual at increased risk of stroke. So, if you have migraine with aura you must not use any of the CHCs for contraception, because this will potentially further increase your risk of stroke. See Chapter 2 for a description of aura, but talk to your doctor if you are unsure. If you develop your first aura while you are using a CHC, you must stop the CHC immediately. Get medical advice and use an alternative contraception method. Many of the progestogen-only methods are actually more effective at preventing pregnancy than CHCs.

Women with migraine without aura can use CHCs provided that they do not have other risk factors for stroke. These include heavy smoking, high blood pressure, high cholesterol, diabetes and obesity. You can continue to use all of the anti-migraine medications, including triptans, which do not appear to increase the risk further. Only ergots are not recommended. Your doctor will advise you if you use topiramate – it may reduce the effectiveness of some contraceptive pills.

Progestogen-only contraception

This type of hormonal contraception includes progestogen-only pills (the 'mini-pill') taken daily and injections given every three months. Alternatively, an implant under the skin or a device inserted directly into the womb (intra-uterine) will release progestogen slowly and may be kept in place for several years.

We have evidence that progestogen-only contraceptives are not associated with an increased risk of stroke. They can be used if you have migraine, including migraine with aura.

Effect of hormonal contraception on headaches and migraine

Headaches and migraines may initially worsen during the first cycles of use but then improve with each cycle. Three months is a usual minimum, and headaches will often completely settle by six months. If they persist on CHCs, then changing to a progestogen-only method may help.

Headaches and migraine typically occur during the hormone-free interval of the standard CHC pill regimen (21 days on/seven days off). The likely cause is oestrogen withdrawal – similar to that occurring in menstrual migraine. Some women may be sensitive to any drops in oes-trogen. To avoid this, your doctor may recommend 'tricycling' (taking three pill packets back to back without a pill-free break). You then have only five withdrawal bleeds – and hopefully only five migraines – instead of 13 each year. Some specialists recommend continuous pill use (extended duration) without a break at all, which may benefit menstrual migraine. Although there appear to be no health benefits of having the hormonal withdrawal bleed, we currently don't know whether the con-tinuous use strategy carries any long-term risks.

Non-hormonal contraception

Non-hormonal contraception includes coils, which do not release hor-mones, and barrier methods such as condoms and caps. They do not normally affect headache and migraine. However, the copper coil can increase bleeding, which may be associated with headache.

Tips for coping with hormonal headaches

- Keep a diary for at least three months to look for links between headaches and hormones. Include headaches, migraines and menstrual periods. Write down each time you take hormonal treatments (e.g. hormonal contraceptives and hormone replacement therapy) and any menopausal symptoms.

- Take time to get some exercise, adopt a regular sleep pattern and eat a balanced diet. Generally feeling healthier may mean that hormone fluctuations are less likely to trigger headaches.
- If simple strategies are not effective, if symptoms are very severe, or if your periods become heavy or painful or you have bleeding in between them, contact your doctor.
- Be informed about your body and try to become more aware of your own hormone cycles. By being 'in tune', you are more likely to cope with the headaches.
- Remember non-hormonal triggers. By reducing these first, sometimes a hormonal headache may be avoided altogether.
- If you decide to use hormonal treatments, give them a proper trial. It takes your body at least three months to adjust to additional hormones.
- Some hormone treatments have side effects of headaches, particularly with initial use. In a headache-prone woman, this can feel like a disaster. Don't expect too much too soon and hopefully you will feel the benefits when the headaches settle.

14

Headaches, pregnancy and breastfeeding

Having a baby is a special time but it can be overwhelming. With so much to think about, concerns about headaches can be an additional strain. Will my headache affect my chances of having a baby? What will happen to my headache when I am pregnant? I've just found out I'm pregnant – will headache medications have harmed my baby? Can I breastfeed and treat my headache? This chapter addresses these questions and offers ways to cope with headache before, during and after pregnancy.

The information is mainly related to migraine, but if you have tension-type headache, the advice is still relevant. If you have cluster headache then you are likely to be under the care of a specialist headache doctor. Some drug strategies should be stopped before you conceive and others started or continued in pregnancy under close medical supervision. Seek advice before you become pregnant if possible.

Effect of headaches on having a baby

There is no evidence so far that women with primary headaches who are otherwise healthy are less likely to conceive. There is also no suggestion that you are at greater risk than the general population of miscarriage, stillbirth, birth defects or problems with growth and development of the baby. There is an increased risk of pre-eclampsia and eclampsia in women with migraine, especially if they are overweight. Midwives and doctors monitor all pregnant women very carefully for these potentially serious conditions, by checking blood pressure and urine protein levels.

What happens to headaches in pregnancy?

Elizabeth, 41
'I have suffered from severe migraine with my periods for since I was a teenager. The only time I ever had any respite was during my two pregnancies. It was bliss!'

For many women, especially those with migraine, headaches may be less of a problem during pregnancy. Around two thirds of women who have migraine notice improvement during pregnancy, particularly after the first trimester (three months). Some women notice no change and a few get worse. Improvement is more likely with migraine without aura, which is linked to periods and can last during breastfeeding until menstruation returns. The reasons why this is so are unclear, because many changes occur in a woman's body during pregnancy. It may be related to higher or more stable levels of the hormone oestrogen, changes in blood sugar levels and higher levels of endorphins – the body's natural painkillers.

Non-hormonally related migraine and migraine with aura are less likely to improve. If women develop migraine for the first time in pregnancy, it is more commonly migraine with aura and may be just the aura without the headache. (See Chapter 2.) If you develop aura and/or any new headache while you are pregnant, it is important that you talk to your doctor, who will be able to reassure you or conduct further tests.

Tips for coping with headaches and preparing for pregnancy

Planning for pregnancy is a good time to think about your current headache coping strategies and optimize your general health before conceiving. This is particularly important if you use drug treatments, because these are more likely to affect a developing baby during the first three months, often before you know you are pregnant. Here are some ways to prepare.

- Ensure that your lifestyle is as healthy as possible. This will help you and your baby, and it may help with your headaches. This includes giving up smoking and alcohol, taking regular exercise and losing (or putting on) weight if necessary.
- Eat a balanced diet. Ensure that meals are regular. Avoid triggering a migraine by keeping blood sugar levels stable and avoiding dehydration.
- Take a vitamin supplement recommended for pregnancy that includes folic acid and iron.
- Try non-drug therapies to help headache. Migraine may improve during pregnancy and breastfeeding, and drug treatments – particularly preventatives – may no longer be required.
- Discuss with your doctor all medications you are taking, including

herbal and over-the-counter treatments. Some may need to be stopped or changed.

- Limit drug treatments for headache symptoms to the first two weeks of your menstrual cycle if possible, because this is when you are least likely to be pregnant. These are the days of your period and approximately the next ten days before you ovulate (release an egg from your ovaries).
- Medication over-use headache should be tackled before trying for a baby, if possible.

Coping without drugs during pregnancy and breastfeeding

There is a perception that any headache treatment that does not involve prescription drugs is milder, natural and therefore safer for your baby. It can be difficult to decide what is best for you and your baby. Ultimately, what you choose to do is a personal decision.

Physical and complementary therapies

Jane, 33

'I was keen to avoid all drugs when I was expecting my first baby so I tried a course of acupuncture. I told my acupuncturist that I was six weeks pregnant. My migraines stopped shortly after starting and so did my dreadful morning sickness. I felt well throughout the rest of my pregnancy and was really pleased that I did not need to take my usual migraine drugs.'

Physical and complementary therapies for headaches and migraine may be effective for some women while they are pregnant or breast-feeding. Simple techniques such as hot or cold packs on the head can be helpful, as can yoga, relaxation techniques, deep breathing and biofeedback. Acupuncture and massage may be useful under the care of qualified practitioners. Tell your practitioner that you are pregnant or breastfeeding, because this may influence the treatment. For example, some of the essential oils are not used in aromatherapy massage on pregnant women. The benefits of non-drug approaches may last beyond pregnancy and breastfeeding.

Herbal treatments and vitamins

Many women wonder about using herbs for migraine prevention during pregnancy. Unfortunately, these cannot be recommended. There's less information about safety for these products than for prescription medicines, which go through tough evaluation before they become widely available.

Of the herbs that have shown some effectiveness in migraine prevention, neither feverfew nor butterbur is recommended in pregnancy. Feverfew may cause bleeding problems and so should not be used. Ginger is reported to be helpful for treating morning sickness and may also be useful for the sickness associated with migraine attacks, although data are limited.

Vitamins B_2 and B_6 are sometimes used for migraine prevention, but the high doses required are not recommended during pregnancy and breastfeeding. A standard multi-vitamin preparation is a better option and may promote general health and well being.

If you decide to use herbs or diet supplements, minimize any possible risk. Read labels, purchase from a reputable source, use small amounts and ask your doctor, midwife or therapist for advice. New evidence on what is unsafe may become available. Evidence on what is actually safe is unlikely, because large-scale scientific clinical trials to provide evidence are not widely done.

Drug treatments for headache during pregnancy and breastfeeding

Sally, 28

'I was one of the unlucky ones as my migraines got much worse when I was pregnant. I was using paracetamol and my GP [general practitioner] recommended a low dose of beta-blockers for migraine prevention. I was worried about taking a tablet every day, but my attacks improved and I felt much better in myself. He explained that no medicines are "safe" in pregnancy but for the ones I was using, we did not have reason to think that they would harm the baby.'

Because it is unethical to carry out research trials to determine the safety of drugs in pregnancy and breastfeeding, we can't be certain how drugs will affect the growth and development of the baby. Information we have about safety is mostly circumstantial and very limited.

Your doctor and/or midwife will advise you on how to make the best decision for you and your baby. If you have been taking medications for migraine and discover that you are pregnant, then it is unlikely that you will have caused any harm. Even if drugs not recommended in pregnancy were accidentally taken, this in itself is not a medical reason to terminate the pregnancy. However, once you know that you are pregnant it is always best to use as few drugs as possible and in the lowest effective doses.

The lack of clinical trial data doesn't mean that you should not use medications at all, but it does mean that you need to make an informed choice by weighing up the risks and the benefits. Your doctor will carefully assess this for both you and your baby before he or she prescribes your treatment. Some cases of debilitating, severe headache may require effective treatment to avoid associated poor eating, poor sleep, dehydration and increased stress. All of these are unhealthy for both mother and baby.

Caution is still essential while breastfeeding because although medications are less restricted than during pregnancy, the drugs may pass from breast milk to the baby. This happens more readily with some drugs than with others.

Drugs to treat headache symptoms

Generally, paracetamol is the drug of choice. It may be used throughout pregnancy and breastfeeding because it does not appear to affect the baby. It is best taken in soluble form, ideally with something to eat. Aspirin is not usually recommended because it can cause problems with bleeding. It should always be avoided completely during the last three months of pregnancy and during breastfeeding.

Non-steroidal anti-inflammatory drugs are occasionally suggested in early pregnancy, but they should not be used during the last trimester. They may be used in breastfeeding with caution. The doses are kept low and repeated only if necessary. Occasional low doses of codeine in combined painkillers are probably not harmful during pregnancy and breastfeeding, but data are limited. Because it can aggravate nausea, codeine is not recommended for migraine.

Ergotamine should not be used in pregnancy because it can increase the risk of miscarriage. It is not recommended in breastfeeding because it may stop milk production.

Triptans in pregnancy and breastfeeding

Healthcare professionals are encouraged to report pregnancy outcomes to databases of safety information on triptans used to treat migraine. The evidence, so far mainly from the sumatriptan pregnancy registry, is reassuring but still limited. The number of women is small, data reporting is biased and there is little information from the later stages of pregnancy. Therefore, the use of triptans in pregnancy cannot be recommended. Data suggest that sumatriptan can be used while breast-feeding but that you should allow at least 12 hours between taking the drug and breastfeeding. Because there are fewer data for the other triptans, the current advice is to exercise caution. In practice this means waiting for 24 hours before breastfeeding if you have used almotriptan, eletriptan, frovatriptan, naratriptan, rizatriptan or zolmitriptan for migraine.

Anti-sickness medications

Domperidone, buclizine, chlorpromazine, metoclopramide and prochlorperazine are not reported to cause harm during pregnancy and breastfeeding. Discuss with your doctor which is the best one for you. During breastfeeding, domperidone – which can increase milk produc-tion – is preferred to metoclopramide.

Drugs to prevent headache symptoms

Migraine often improves during pregnancy, so this is a good time to consider stopping daily preventatives. Occasionally, preventative drug strategies are commenced if headaches are frequent and severe or to reduce the amount of symptomatic medications.

The recommended preventative is the beta-blocker propanolol at the lowest effective dose. Although this has been widely used, it is usually stopped a few days before delivery because it can slow the baby's heart rate, cause low blood sugar levels in the baby and affect contractions. Other preventatives such as low doses of amitriptyline and pizotifen are sometimes used. In the absence of epilepsy, the anti-epileptics are not recommended because some may cause birth defects.

After delivery and breastfeeding

About 30–40 per cent of women have a migraine or headache within a few days of delivery. This can be very severe and may be due to hormonal changes such as a drop in oestrogen levels and endorphin levels returning to normal. Dehydration, extreme exhaustion and low blood sugar levels may also be significant. Their need for effective drug treatments for headache can make some women reluctant to start breastfeeding. Others give up prematurely for the same reason. However, headaches often settle down again, so if you do want to breastfeed it would be a shame not to. Although it can take a little while to establish, breastfeeding is highly recommended.

Tips for coping with headaches during pregnancy and breastfeeding

- If your headaches stay the same or get worse, this doesn't mean that there is anything wrong. Speak to your doctor for reassurance.
- You should always see your doctor if you develop any *new* headaches or unusual accompanying symptoms. He or she may run tests if necessary.
- Don't forget to avoid your usual headache triggers. Take extra care to avoid becoming dehydrated and eat little and often. This can be difficult if morning sickness is causing low blood sugar and dehydration. Ginger in tea or biscuits may be helpful. When you have had your baby and routines change, continue to avoid these triggers.
- Avoid over-tiredness, which is a migraine trigger. This is important during the first and last trimesters (three months) of pregnancy. It can be impossible with a new baby, but aim for a regular sleep pattern as soon as you can. Accept offers of help and get into a routine that allows you the rest that you need.
- Minimize additional stress if you can. Take exercise, have a massage, do things you enjoy and order shopping online. Don't feel guilty about making things easier for yourself. Avoiding headaches is better than treating them, but especially when options are more limited.
- Make time to continue with helpful non-drug treatments once you have had your baby.
- If you need medication for headaches, ask your doctor about those that are considered low risk during pregnancy and breastfeeding.
- Medication over-use can occur in pregnancy. Be aware of this possibility if you are regularly treating headache symptoms on three days a week.
- Anticipate the possibility of a severe headache in the early days after delivery and have potential treatments available. Discuss options with your healthcare team in advance.
- Try not to give up breastfeeding if you have headaches during the first few days after delivery. If you suffered from hormonally related headaches before pregnancy and they improved during pregnancy, they may settle down in the first few weeks. (Often when you stop breastfeeding and periods return, the headaches

come back, but by that time you will have more treatment
options anyway.)

- Keep your baby's exposure to drugs to a minimum by considering
  the time at which you take your medication. Dosing immediately
  after breastfeeding or waiting until after the last feed of the day
  when the baby has a longer sleep can make a difference.
- Express and throw away breast milk while you are treating a
  migraine attack with non-recommended medications, such
  as triptans. Even though you feel unwell, it is worth doing to
  encourage ongoing milk production. It also helps to prevent your
  breasts becoming engorged and uncomfortable.
- Keep a supply of expressed breast milk in the freezer for use
  when you are unable to breastfeed, having taken medications.
  Alternatively, have a supply of formula milk ready to use.

15

Headaches, menopause and HRT

Sarah, 48
'My migraines got much worse in my early forties and have controlled my life in recent years. I can't wait for the menopause to arrive because I am hoping that the migraines will stop along with the periods. My mother's headaches got better after the menopause and I hope mine will too.'

The menopause

The menopause is the time of your last menstrual period and marks the end of your reproductive life. The average age for menopause is around 51 years, but it can happen from any time between 40 and 60. Medically, the definition of menopause is no periods for 12 consecutive months after the age of 50 or for two years under the age of 50. Until menopause is confirmed you should still use adequate contraception.

The perimenopause

The perimenopause is the time of change that leads to the menopause. Your hormone cycles begin to change and become disrupted. Menstrual periods are more erratic – sometimes closer together and at other times further apart. They may also become heavier and more painful. This time, the 'climacteric' or simply 'the change of life', can last up to 20 years.

Symptoms of the perimenopause

Hormone changes and fluctuations can be accompanied by many symptoms. Sometimes severe, they are mainly due to low oestrogen levels. These include more frequent and severe headaches and migraines, which are often linked to periods. Other troublesome symptoms can include:

- irregular periods – often shorter cycles and then missed periods;
- hot flushes and night sweats;
- mood changes – irritability, anxiety and depression;
- dry skin, hair and eyes;
- poor memory and concentration;
- weight gain;
- sexual problems – dryness and/or itching of the vagina, painful intercourse and loss of interest in sex;
- loss of energy and sleep disruption;
- muscle and joint pain;
- urinary problems – infections, urgent need to urinate and leakage when coughing or running; and
- heart palpitations.

The presence of some of these symptoms in a woman over 40 is enough to confirm the perimenopause, and so blood tests are not usually necessary.

Types of headaches around the menopause

Although migraine is strongly influenced by female hormones, not all headaches occurring around the menopause are migrainous in nature and tension-type headache can occur too. Fortunately, cluster headache is not only less common in women but it also seems to improve with increasing age. There appears to be no association with female hormones. Daily headaches made worse by daily medications can be a particular problem at this time of life.

Change in headaches around the menopause

If you have headaches related to oestrogen withdrawal, then you should be able to expect an improvement after menopause. This is because oestrogen levels decline in the first year after menopause and then remain low and stable. Although, we can't reliably predict what will happen, there is a good chance that migraine will improve. However, it can take between two and five years after menopause for the hormones to settle down and cease to be a trigger.

One study found that almost two thirds of women who had history of migraine noticed an improvement after menopause was established. Around ten per cent had worse headaches and 25 per cent did not notice any change. Another study found 53 per cent less migraine without aura in postmenopausal women. Migraine with aura may change less after menopause than migraine without aura. Interestingly, time since menopause was more important than having migraines with menstruation previously. This implies that it isn't just the reduced influence of hormonal factors that improves migraine, but retirement and reduced stress may also be involved. Neck stiffness or other ailments as you get older may contribute to worsening headaches.

Coping with headaches around the menopause

Despite the menopause being a natural change to your body, headaches and migraines are part of a range of menopausal symptoms that add up to make you feel really unwell. This has a negative impact on your whole life. Some women are not badly affected but others are severely incapacitated physically or mentally, or both. Recognizing this is important, and there are ways to improve how you feel that do not involve hormone replacement therapy (HRT). The better you feel overall, the better you will cope with your headaches. Unfortunately, if your menopause symptoms are troublesome, then you are more likely to be prone to them.

Don't tackle menopause symptoms in isolation and remember measures to cope with headaches too! Migraine triggers add up. If you are exhausted from broken sleep due to night sweats, then this tiredness could trigger an attack, regardless of your hormones. If many symptoms are combining to make you feel awful, sometimes an improvement in just one symptom can help.

Coping without drugs

Despite little scientific evidence, around half of women report that self-help and complementary measures benefit their menopausal symptoms. Although less effective than HRT, they are worth trying, especially if you don't wish to use HRT or can't use it for health reasons.

Exercise

Evidence suggests that aerobic exercise like swimming can be beneficial for menopausal symptoms, and all weight bearing exercise is good for maintaining strong bones. Exercise may be helpful for your headaches, but eat enough and don't become dehydrated or this can be a trigger. Get into a sensible routine – overdoing it every now and then will make you feel worse.

Plant oestrogens (phytoestrogens)

These are also called isoflavones and are obtained from soy and red clover. This way of supplementing oestrogens may be helpful and is being researched. We don't have any long-term safety data. You should not use isoflavones if you have a condition in which oestrogen is not recommended (e.g. breast cancer). So far, data on whether they can help or trigger migraine is conflicting.

Diet and supplements

Try to eat a healthy balanced diet. Hot flushes and night sweats may be reduced both in number and severity by reducing alcohol and caffeine. If you cut down on tea and coffee, do it gradually to avoid a caffeine withdrawal headache. Avoid headache tablets containing caffeine.

We have no evidence that supplements of vitamin E, vitamin C, selenium or evening primrose oil bring particular benefits. Although evening primrose oil may help with breast tenderness, it can cause headache as a side effect.

Agnus castus may help symptoms of premenstrual syndrome, but there is no evidence for its ability to help with menopausal symptoms. Dong quai, *Ginkgo biloba*, ginseng, St John's wort and black cohosh have all been widely used. Some women experience improvement but some of these are known to interact with medications and may have side effects, including headaches.

Complementary therapies

Although scientific studies have not demonstrated significant improvements and more long-term trials are needed, some women have found benefit from acupuncture and homeopathy. Tell your therapist about all your headaches and symptoms.

Ingrid, 53

'My migraines became more frequent as I got older. Broken sleep from night sweats made me really tired and I'm sure that made things worse. I felt like I could get a migraine at any time, all the time. I realized I would have to take more care of myself – I'd been too busy before! I started using red clover. I tried to eat regular meals, have more water instead of coffee and get more early nights. After about six months I felt much better. I think the red clover and a few changes made a difference to get me through a difficult time. I had my last period two years ago and hardly ever have a migraine now.'

Prescription drugs (non-hormone replacement therapy)

There are several alternatives to HRT, and some may have a positive influence on headaches and migraines.

Selective serotonin re-uptake inhibitors

Selective serotonin re-uptake inhibitors (also known as SSRIs) include fluoxetine and paroxetine and are widely used as anti-depressants. They have also been shown to help severe sweating and flushing symptoms associated with menopause and may help migraine and headaches. Another type of anti-depressant called venlafaxine can be helpful. To minimise the likelihood of side effects, doses are usually lower than for depression. Headaches can worsen in initial months, so don't give up too soon.

Gabapentin

This anti-epileptic has been found to reduce symptoms of flushes, aches and pains in many menopausal women. Although it is used in migraine prevention, there is no good scientific evidence of it working well. Doses are started low and increased gradually to minimize side effects, which can include dizziness and sedation.

Clonidine

Used to control blood pressure, clonidine may be helpful in reducing hot flushes in some women. Although it is licensed for migraine prevention, there are other more effective preventative treatments available. Side effects include dizziness, sedation and worsening of any depression.

Hormone replacement therapy and headaches

HRT is not recommended if your only menopause problem is headache. It is far better to use standard headache strategies, and for many women they are enough to cope well. However, if you are battling with severe menopausal symptoms in addition to your headaches, then HRT may be worth considering. It does not suit all women, but for others it can transform their life.

What is hormone replacement therapy?

HRT remains the best treatment and can improve menopausal symptoms for over 80 per cent of women. It is prescribed with the aim of balancing hormones. The main component is oestrogen, because many of the troublesome symptoms of the menopause are believed to be due to low oestrogen levels. If you haven't had a hysterectomy, you will also need to take a progestogen. This reduces the risk of oestrogen causing thickening and over-stimulation of the endometrium (lining of the womb). This is important because otherwise cancerous changes can develop. HRT doesn't always suppress the normal menstrual cycle, nor is it contraceptive.

Migraine, health risks and hormone replacement therapy

HRT has had bad press in recent years for all women, not just those who have migraine. There have been concerns over long-term safety, risks of breast and other cancers, heart disease, blood clots and strokes.

Although there are few data, no evidence so far suggests that having migraine with or without aura poses an additional health risk. This means provided that all your other risk factors have been taken into account by your doctor, having migraine alone will not stop you from taking HRT. You can continue your migraine treatments, including triptans and prevention medications, while you are using HRT.

Effect of hormone replacement therapy on headache and migraine

Few clinical studies have considered the impact of HRT on non-migraine headache and results have provided conflicting information. Some women notice an improvement, others no change and some find that their headaches get worse.

In theory, if you have hormonally related migraine then you should benefit from the stabilizing of oestrogen levels with HRT. Although some women do benefit greatly, this doesn't always happen. Data from questionnaire studies suggest that using HRT can aggravate migraines in some women, and this seems more likely if your migraines worsened during the perimenopause. We need more research on who might develop headache problems on HRT. There is some suggestion that if you had premenstrual syndrome then you may be more prone to the headache side effects of HRT.

In practice, we can't predict whether you will benefit or not. It is trial and error to find the HRT that suits you best. If your menopause symptoms are severe and affecting your life, find out whether HRT is an option and discuss the pros and cons with your doctor.

Best hormone replacement therapy for headaches

Joan, 50

'I had terrible hot flushes, which were so embarrassing. At night the sweats drenched me and I often needed to change the sheets. I was getting tired and depressed. Although the HRT tablets my GP [general practitioner] prescribed worked wonders with the flushes and sweats, I got severe migraines all the time. The GP switched me to using HRT patches you wear on your skin. This suited me much better. The headaches have settled and I feel more like myself again.'

Despite a lack of clinical trial data, there are clues about which regimens and types of HRT may be less aggravating for headaches. Some types of HRT may even benefit hormonally triggered migraine. The aim of any HRT treatment is to reduce symptoms at the lowest possible dose of hormones.

Oestrogen component

Oestrogen fluctuations can be a trigger for migraine. Gels or skin patches, which provide more stable oestrogen levels, are better than tablets. Also, continuous HRT is less likely to cause oestrogen 'withdrawal' migraines than the cyclical regimens.

Oestrogen in too high a dose can cause migraine aura. Tell your doctor if you notice any changes in your headaches or accompanying symptoms. After other medical conditions are excluded, headache and aura symptoms are often resolved by lowering the dose or changing the way that it is taken.

Progestogen component

Patches, implants and injections are less likely to cause headaches because, unlike tablets, they maintain more stable levels of progestogen. Continuous progestogen is preferable to cyclical regimens, which are known to aggravate headaches.

Side effects of progestogen include headache and symptoms similar to those of premenstrual syndrome. These may be improved by changing the progestogen type or way in which it is taken. It is important that you do not stop taking the progestogen, which is needed to protect the lining of your womb.

We have no data on which type of progestogen may be better for women with headaches. Some women prefer progesterone derivatives to testosterone derivatives. The Mirena® intra-uterine system is a newer, well tolerated way to take progestogen. It is contraceptive and can be helpful for women with migraine. Because it provides protection to the womb, your doctor can adjust the oestrogen dose and formulation to meet your needs.

Tips for coping with headaches around the menopause

- Keep a diary of your headaches and migraines to assess the effect of treatment strategies.
- Don't forget about non-hormonal triggers.
- Aim to optimize symptomatic headache treatments and consider preventatives if headaches increase.
- Report any treatment side effects and changes in health to your doctor. If you are unwell for any reason, this may make headaches worse.
- If you decide to use HRT, then give it a proper trial. It takes time for your body to adjust to hormones, so ideally use it for at least three months. Headache and migraine may worsen during this time before an improvement is noticed.

16
Helping yourself

Accepting that you have a predisposition to headaches is part of coping. The next part is doing something about it. Although medications and therapies have their place, you must decide to help yourself as well. This doesn't have to be difficult because small changes in your lifestyle can make big differences. It is about you taking ownership of the situation and not being a passive recipient of treatments and drugs. This chapter outlines very simple but effective ideas to help you cope better.

Learn about your headache

Reading a simple headache book like this one is a good start. There is a lot of information on headaches available on the internet, but you need to be sure that it is from a reliable source. Some websites only want to sell you a product. Always be selective and highly critical.

Research has shown us that people with headaches don't just want pain relief – they need to understand more about their headache. This is an important part of coping. If your headache is severe, being reassured and understanding that it is a proper neurological disorder is essential. You need to feel that it isn't just you who feels like this and to understand that you are not going mad. Because those of us with headaches may not often go to our doctor (and doctors are not always interested in headaches anyway), it is down to us to be informed and to ask questions about our headaches. We can then find out how to help ourselves, and what might be available to assist us. Think of this as ongoing – new ideas and treatments are always being developed.

Join a headache organization or group

Joining an organization is useful to learn about headache and keep up to date with new treatments and research. (See Useful addresses, at the end of this book.) The organizations have informative websites (even for non-members), newsletters and information days. They can tell you where to find headache clinics if you need more support. Information on finding or starting a local self-help group is also available. Some people find it helpful to talk to others who understand the impact of headaches on their lives and families. This isn't true for everyone but could be worth thinking about. People with cluster headache in particular may find it enlightening to talk to others. Because it is rare, they are unlikely to have met anyone else with it and can feel isolated.

Keep a headache diary

You do not need to keep a diary indefinitely – just while you are reviewing your headaches and treatments. Be honest and note *all* headaches and *all* medications. Include over-the-counter painkillers and not just triptans for migraine. For cluster headache, record even the 'little niggles' before the bout starts. Understanding how they build up could provide valuable information on when to start preventative treatment next time. In short, everything counts!

Why keep a diary?

A diary is useful to track what is happening. It can help you, your doctor and your therapist to see whether strategies or lifestyle changes are having a positive effect. By considering 'before and after' headache patterns, this can be more obvious. If you didn't write it down, it is difficult to remember what was happening a few months ago. Sometimes when headaches have improved, but not gone altogether, you can forget what they were like. Remember that improvement takes various forms. It might not be headache frequency that improves – it could be severity, duration or perhaps taking fewer tablets and having less side effects.

Attack diaries provide information on frequency of headache and migraine, type and time when medication is taken, amount of medication taken, patterns at weekends, time the headaches started, changes in headache over time and the relationship to periods in women. All of this is helpful for checking diagnoses and optimizing treatments.

Trigger diaries for migraine encourage you to record food, drink, emotional state, sleep, daily activities and, in women, periods. This is to look for patterns, connections and possibly triggers to avoid. Don't get too obsessed with keeping these diaries other than for a short time – usually these triggers are fairly obvious.

Obtaining a diary

You can devise your own diary – whatever makes sense to you and is easy to keep. Various diaries are available from headache organizations and from the internet. (See Useful addresses at the end of this book.) You need to find one that is right for you. You can download the simple annual and monthly diaries we use at the City of London Migraine Clinic (<www.migraineclinic.org.uk>). These attack diaries are simple to fill in (even children can do it) and provide information at a glance.

Recognize and manage triggers

The relevance of triggers varies between headaches and individuals. If there are trigger factors for your headache, then it is up to you to avoid the ones that you can do something about. This can be alcohol for cluster headache or the build up of stress and muscle tension for tension-type headache.

Many triggers can affect migraine. Assessing and avoiding triggers requires commitment and an understanding of how they build up to tip you over your migraine threshold. One recent patient at the City of London Migraine Clinic had two consecutive months of severe menstrually related migraine, lasting several days. She kept a detailed diary and we were surprised to observe that each one coincided with a business trip. It transpired that the short trips were so pressurized that she was completely out of her usual routine and had little time to eat or sleep properly. We suggested travelling at a different time in her cycle and not to forget about the non-menstrual triggers, which can add up. At her follow-up visit the menstrually related migraine still occurred, but it was more manageable.

Be prepared and get organized

Although this may seem obvious, you must be prepared to prevent headaches and to tackle them quickly. Depending on your lifestyle, this can take some organizing. It means renewing prescriptions before they run out; having treatments in your bag, jacket or car; and remembering them even if you change your routine. I had a severe migraine because I was away at a conference (embarrassingly, a headache one), didn't drink enough water, didn't eat regularly *and* left my medication in my hotel room, because I had a different bag with me.

If you often wake with migraine in the middle of the night, have your medications by your bedside with a glass of water. Jennifer, one of our patients at the Clinic, uses tiny plastic pots with lids. She has her combination of tablets for each dose in each pot. Small pots like this are just the right size to keep ready for use by your bed but also in your bag or pocket. This saves valuable time because early treatment can stop the attack taking hold. Likewise, you need to be organized in your prevention by carrying a drink of water and planning to eat regularly. If you have migraine, being late for a meal by just an hour can trigger an attack. Plan ahead and carry a snack to be on the safe side.

If you have cluster headache you may not want to think about the next bout, but it makes sense to be prepared. Always have a current prescription and supply of your treatments so that you can start them immediately. Waiting days for a doctor's appointment causes unnecessary delay when you need pain relief.

Use over-the-counter treatments carefully

Over-the-counter treatments include a range of painkiller medications, herbs and supplements. These can be helpful to cope with headaches. Be cautious if you are using medications on ten to 15 days per month because over-use can perpetuate the cycle of headache. Additionally, various gadgets and aids such as cooling strips for headache are available. Choosing to buy over-the-counter is a key part of coping and being in control of your headache. You can make choices about what you use and might find something that brings you relief. However, be wary of any promises of cure. If something sounds too good, then it probably is.

The pharmacist

Your pharmacist can advise on coping, over-the-counter and prescription medications, and whether you need medical help. Always ask to speak with the pharmacist directly – not the counter assistants. You can purchase the anti-migraine drug sumatriptan over-the-counter in the UK by completing a form and discussing it with the pharmacist.

Take part in research

Scientific research projects on headache and clinical trials on drugs and treatments provide evidence that can increase our understanding. They help us to discover new and better ways of treating and preventing headaches. There is still so much to learn, so do find out about research and consider participating. The headache organizations advertise when volunteers are required or you can enquire directly.

It is potentially an opportunity to help yourself and others in the future. You may try new treatments before anyone else and have access to expert doctors. Even if the study doesn't help you directly, the information is still valuable.

Don't let placebos (dummy treatments) put you off taking part, because the chances of receiving one are often low. We need placebos to ensure treatments really work and are better than what we have already. Our brains release chemicals to improve pain on suggestion alone. A strong placebo effect may account for why some medications and therapies work for headache. Outside of research trials this doesn't matter, as long as it does no harm and you feel better!

17

Looking after yourself

Looking after your health is essential and is very easy to forget with the fast pace of modern life or if your headache dominates your health concerns. This chapter covers some of the issues that can have an impact on your health and could influence your headaches.

General health

Very simply, if your general health is poor and you are prone to headaches of any type, then you will not cope well. Poor health could contribute to making headaches worse too. A balanced diet, plenty of water and getting enough sleep will all help.

Exercise

You should exercise regularly. Research suggests that inactive people are more likely to have headaches. Exercise is particularly helpful for tension-type headache and need not provoke migraine if sensible precautions are taken. (See Chapter 19.)

Smoking

The connection with smoking and headaches is unknown. It can be a trigger for headache in a few people (even passive smoking), and those with cluster headache are often smokers. Smoking increases the risk of stroke and diseases of the heart and blood vessels. If you have migraine, then smoking increases your risk of stroke further. If you develop heart and or circulatory problems due to smoking, you will be unable to use triptans for migraine because they constrict blood vessels. Smoking also increases risk of many cancers, not just lung cancer.

Give up smoking if you can. It is the single best thing you can do for your general health and there is help available. (See Useful addresses at the end of this book.)

Eye strain

Surprisingly eye problems rarely cause headaches. Have regular check ups with your optician if you wear glasses or contact lenses or if you sense a problem with your eyes or sight. Opticians can check your overall eye health and detect potentially serious causes of headache. If you have migraine with aura, the visual disturbances are associated with changes in brain chemistry – not problems with your eyes. However, if you have eye strain, this may act as an additional trigger for migraine in some people, so it is worth eliminating.

Dental problems

Visiting your dentist may not seem very relevant to headache, but lingering gum infections or other teeth problems can cause head pain directly. They can also lower your threshold for developing headache and migraine, and so regular visits and good dental hygiene are important.

Medical problems

Although self-help plays a major role in managing many types of headache, you should recognize when you need medical help. That isn't just for headache (see Chapter 1), but also if there is something else wrong with you. If you have another illness or condition that is uncontrolled, then your headaches may worsen. If you have symptoms that seem minor but don't improve, visit your doctor. Headaches and migraine can improve dramatically when other conditions are recognized and controlled, including injuries; infections; back, neck, teeth, jaw, sinus or eye problems; period problems; depression and anxiety; fibromyalgia; thyroid diseases; insomnia; and even constipation.

Psychological health

Looking after psychological health might seem strange, because headaches are real disorders and are not 'all in the head'. However, in ways we don't fully understand, emotional factors play a part in headaches and how we deal with them. It has been suggested that people with migraine have certain personality types and are very driven and perfectionist. Although not proven, it isn't very helpful because we can't easily change our personalities! Here are some ideas about trying to feel better.

Help from family and friends

People offer help, but we don't always accept it and struggle on. Think about 'lightening your load', not just when you are experiencing debilitating headaches and can't do anything, but the rest of the time too.

Organize family routines for household chores and cover from friends. Children are often surprisingly good at dealing with responsibility when a parent is unwell. Encourage everyone in the family to help in their own little ways.

Gather extra support so that everything continues if you are stopped in your tracks by a headache. By sharing everyday pressures and not allowing them to escalate, you may raise your threshold for developing headaches and particularly migraine. You don't have to feel guilty, because you know that you pull your weight when you don't have a headache. It isn't about giving into headaches – it is about living with headaches.

This of course is easier said than done. Lyn, a patient at the City of London Migraine Clinic, told me that losing a leg is so visible that everyone can imagine what you might be experiencing. How different it is for people with migraine – everyone thinks it's just a bad headache and they have no idea how debilitating it is. This is part of the hidden problem of headaches – no one really understands what is happening, unless you explain and allow them to help.

Personal relationships

Lyn estimates that she loses about 20 per cent of her life to debilitating migraine attacks and couldn't get by without the support of her husband. Don't underestimate the impact of headaches on both you and your partner. You need his or her support. It is best to be open and communicate your problems and needs so that you deal with your headache together. You may feel guilty about letting your partner down if social occasions are missed and if headaches are an intrusion on family life. There may be times when you cannot take your share of the responsibility. This can be worse if you feel you have brought the headache upon yourself. Remember that this isn't true – it is a neurobiological disorder that you have a tendency toward. As long as you are doing your best to deal with your headache, there is nothing more that you (or anyone else) can expect.

Headaches and sex

Dealing with headaches has an impact on all areas of our lives, including our sex life. It is always a joke – even with people who don't have them – that a headache is an excuse not to have sex. It isn't a joke if your headache is affecting this aspect of your life.

Any long-term medical conditions, including headaches, can adversely affect your desire for sex (libido). It is easy for a partner to feel continually rejected and for your relationship to become strained.

Supporting each other and good communication is important to deal with this.

For some people sex can actually cause headaches. They usually occur before or during orgasm. They are more common in men, people with migraine and those with high blood pressure. If you notice this for the first time, you should see your doctor. Occasionally sudden, severe, 'explosive' headaches occurring at orgasm have been associated with a stroke caused by bleeding in the brain. Headaches associated with sexual activity can be due to muscle tension in the head and neck as excitement increases. They don't usually have serious underlying causes, but your doctor should rule these out. Sometimes tests are required and treatments are available.

Relaxation and stress

Learning to relax and cope with stress is important for everyone, but particularly for those with headaches and migraine. If there are sources of stress in your life that you can do something about, then try to deal with them. Tackle issues one step at a time – sometimes just doing something positive is enough to make you feel better.

Take time for yourself, do activities you enjoy and – once in a while – allow yourself time to do nothing at all. You will need to decide to do this, plan time for it to happen and not feel guilty about it. Sometimes the only time people stop is when they are laid up with a headache!

Positive thinking

If thinking positively about headache is too difficult, try at least not to think negatively. Having headaches is a part of your life that you have to deal with, just like anything else. That means finding a treatment that works for you, being confident that you deal with them as best you can and not wasting energy worrying about a headache when you haven't got one. If you are having a bad phase, recognize it as just that – a bad phase that will pass. If treatments are not working as well as they were, find new ones.

Keep taking steps back and thinking about why you might be getting headaches. Is there something you can do about the situation? Has it changed? If you need extra help then get it – see your doctor, therapist or other healthcare professional. You do not have to battle alone. Whatever you do, don't give in. It is essential that you remain in charge of your headaches and that they don't gain control over you. If they do for a while, then try everything you can to shift the balance back again.

Depression

Some people naturally think positively, but others are the opposite and are real worriers. If headaches swamp your life it can be difficult to keep your perspective. If you feel that this is happening to you, then simple self-help measures might not be enough and you might need extra support. Depression readily co-exists with headaches and particularly migraine. If you feel you could be depressed, have a chat with your doctor.

Support at work

Many people don't admit to having headaches, particularly in their work, for fear of discrimination. Unfortunately, there is a stigma attached to having headaches, regardless of whether they are debilitating like migraine or cluster headache – as though they are not a proper illness.

If you can, explain to your colleagues. Having support from your peers and managers is an important part of coping. Explain about your headaches and how you are doing everything you can to help yourself. If you have migraine then ensure your work environment is not unnecessarily triggering your attacks.

A few people are so severely affected by their headache for prolonged periods of time that they are in danger of being overlooked for promotion or even of losing their job. If you need support to deal with your employer, the headache organizations can provide information on how to do this more effectively. (See Useful addresses at the end of this book.) Unfortunately, migraine is long-term but intermittent, so you have a sickness pattern that occupational health departments flag up. Short notice illness puts strain on colleagues who have to cover for you. If you are not getting support at work to do your job effectively and you feel guilty, this can set up a cycle of stress that can perpetuate your headache problem.

18

Diet

If improving headaches were just about removing foods from your diet or adding a particular supplement, it would be so much easier to cope. It isn't that simple – many of you will have already eliminated all sorts of foods from your diet, only to find that your headaches are just the same. This chapter outlines diet considerations that can help. The dietary and herbal supplements most widely used for headaches and migraine are also discussed.

Avoid dehydration

This simple dietary measure can make a difference to the frequency of headaches and migraine. Our bodies are largely made up of water and changes in water balance affect the body's chemistry. For those of us with migraine, dehydration affects excitable nerve cells in our brains, triggering migraine attacks. If we lose more water from our body than we take in, dehydration can occur without us realizing it. I rarely get thirsty and find it difficult to drink enough. If you drink lots of water and still get migraines, don't stop. You are keeping your migraine threshold higher and might otherwise have more attacks. Here are some things to remember.

- Having a drink of water can sometimes stop a headache from developing.
- Don't wait to get thirsty to have a drink, because by then it could be too late.
- Drink plenty of water every day – aim for two litres.
- Keep water convenient and carry a small bottle. It is worth making the effort.
- Caffeine and alcohol are dehydrating, so tea, coffee and alcoholic drinks don't count in the allowance.
- Take extra fluids if you are exercising, the weather is warm or if you are ill with a fever, diarrhoea or vomiting.

Eat enough food

Eating enough is essential for good health and preventing headaches, particularly migraine. Our brain derives energy from glucose (sugar) from our diet and is sensitive to changing blood sugar levels. If they drop (hypoglycaemia) because you have missed or delayed a meal, a migraine can develop quickly.

Lack of food and irregular eating are important triggers for migraine in children and for headaches associated with exercise. It is a major trigger for my migraine. Sometimes it can be less important than others, but remember how migraine triggers can add up. Here is some advice that we give at the City of London Migraine Clinic, which I have found helpful.

- *Eat breakfast* to avoid a migraine attack later in the morning. Fasting overnight and not eating breakfast is too long for those prone to migraine.
- *Eat regularly* to avoid fluctuating blood sugar levels. This should be no longer than four hours, which can be very hard during a busy day. If you are watching your weight eat healthy snacks (e.g. fruit, nuts or seeds). You don't have to eat a lot – little and often will be enough.
- *Eat lunch on time* to avoid a migraine in the late afternoon.
- *Eat food that will sustain you* and experiment with foods and combinations to find what suits you best. Food with a low glycaemic index releases energy more slowly than food with a high index. I have been astonished to discover how I can keep going until lunchtime on a bowl of porridge or muesli, as compared with feeling hungry a couple of hours after eating toast. This is because oat-based cereals have a much lower glycaemic index than bread. Combining carbohydrate with protein in your diet also helps to stabilize blood sugar levels.
- *Eat a snack at bedtime* to avoid the long fast until morning. It can stop migraine waking you during the night. It doesn't have to be too much – another bowl of muesli can work wonders!
- *Eat a varied, balanced diet.* Avoiding too much of any one food group such as sugar, fats, carbohydrates or protein, particularly at one sitting, keeps your blood sugar levels more stable. Reducing sugar, fat, highly processed food and junk food is important for everyone. A healthy diet means dealing with stress better and fighting off illnesses and infections more easily. This makes headaches and migraine much more manageable.

Maintain a normal weight

Being the correct weight for your height isn't just important for your general health. Research suggests that it could help your migraines and headaches too. Now you have another good reason to maintain your healthy weight or lose those extra kilos! Health professionals use a weight/height formula called the body mass index to indicate whether you are in the normal range or overweight or underweight. You can find out more about this from the Patient UK website. (See Useful addresses at the end of this book.)

Having headaches does not appear to be associated with being overweight. However, migraine attacks may be more frequent and increase the more overweight you are. The reasons are unknown. It could be increases in inflammatory substances such as calcitonin gene-related peptide, which are known to be higher in obese people and are implicated in migraine attacks. Higher circulating levels of fats and fatty acids are also inflammatory substances and could be important. One study suggested that a low-fat diet could reduce headaches and the amount of medication required to treat them.

Eliminating specific foods

Many people think that they are 'allergic' to certain foods and that avoiding them will stop headaches, particularly migraines. The body develops antibodies to fight a true allergy, and research has not shown that migraineurs develop this in response to specific foods. Although some people may be sensitive or intolerant to certain foods, they rarely provoke a headache or migraine every time they are consumed. For this reason allergy and intolerance testing specifically for headaches is not usually helpful.

Apart from alcohol and the flavour enhancer monosodium glutamate added to Chinese food, there is little clear research evidence to support eliminating specific foods from your diet to help with headaches. If you find a specific trigger then avoid it, but generally most people find that eliminating foods doesn't help. Anyway, strict elimination diets are difficult to maintain and can make you miserable. More importantly, they may lead to not eating enough, and this is even more likely to trigger headaches and migraine. Additionally, fear and anticipation that something could bring on a migraine attack may be enough to trigger one.

Despite this, the list of postulated potential food triggers is substantial. Here are just a few of them:

- cheese, particularly aged cheeses;
- chocolate;
- citrus fruits;
- pickled foods such as herrings;
- preserved, cured or processed meats such as gammon, bacon, sausage, hot dogs and especially those with nitrites;
- food additives including MSG (monosodium glutamate) and various E numbers;
- artificial sweeteners such as aspartame;
- dried fruits such as raisins, dates and figs;
- peanuts, nuts and seeds;
- smoked or dried fish;
- vinegar;
- fermented products such as soy sauce;
- deep fried food;
- avocados;
- bananas;
- red plums; and
- yeast.

Many of these items contain tyramine, which is naturally found in food from the breakdown of the amino acid tyrosine. The amount varies widely, but it is common in foods that are aged, fermented or have begun to decompose. Tyramine is the likely reason why cheese, chocolate and oranges are always blamed for migraine. Although some people are sensitive, research has not demonstrated a consistent link with tyramine, nitrites or any other food component. At the City of London Migraine Clinic we advise that chocolate is more likely to be a dietary symptom of a migraine attack, rather than a dietary cause. Dr Nat Blau, who founded the Clinic, once told a young boy that he could eat chocolate again, his mother having forbidden it because of migraine. The little lad's smile lit up the consulting room!

It is difficult to know what to do for the best, but some useful tips are provided in the information box.

Tips for identifying foods as a possible trigger for headaches

- Don't stop specific foods or food groups unless you strongly suspect that they contribute to your own headaches or migraines.
- Remember a true sensitivity to a food as a migraine trigger usually causes attacks repeatedly rather than occasionally.

- If you suspect a severe reaction to a food substance, which may include skin rashes and stomach upsets in addition to headache, then consult your doctor. Professional allergy and sensitivity testing may be appropriate.
- A doctor or dietician should monitor any strict diet. Don't commence one without advice if you are pregnant or planning a pregnancy.
- Consider diet triggers in the context of non-dietary triggers and your migraine threshold, rather than in isolation.
- Keep a food and headache diary for two months to see whether there are any recognizable triggers. Remember that the migraine process begins before the headache – so look two or three days *before* it begins.
- If you suspect that a certain food is a trigger, eliminate it for a month and see whether there is a difference. If there isn't, try eating it again and avoid another suspect instead. It is worth being systematic – otherwise you may be depriving yourself of foods in the mistaken belief that they are responsible for headaches.
- Don't make too many changes at once if you want to understand the triggers for your headaches. If you start a new migraine preventative and an elimination diet at the same time, you won't be sure which has helped.

Drink alcohol in moderation

Unlike specific foods, alcohol is a recognized consistent trigger for some headaches, particularly cluster headache. Almost 80 per cent of people with cluster headache reduce their alcohol intake during a cluster bout. The link is less clear with migraine, but migraineurs are much more likely to get a headache triggered by alcohol or succumb to a delayed headache – the hangover. One survey did not find any such sensitivity in those with tension-type headache, and 40 per cent of migraineurs avoided alcohol to avoid triggering migraines.

Type of alcoholic drink and migraine

Red wine and other dark coloured drinks such as whisky, brandy, beer and port are more likely to induce migraine or lead to a hangover headache than white wine or clear spirits such as gin and vodka. Developing a hangover doesn't even have to be related to the amount you drink.

The exact chemicals responsible haven't been identified and sensitivity varies between people and even countries. The French are more likely to get a headache after white wine! Chemicals in dark drinks such as flavonoids, histamine and congeners are possible culprits. Congeners are natural byproducts of alcohol fermentation and give colour, flavour and smell. They could affect blood vessels and encourage the release of inflammatory chemicals to give rise to a migraine.

Headaches and alcohol

Hangover headaches induced by alcohol are delayed, usually occurring when the blood alcohol concentration is falling. They can continue for 24 hours after the level is zero and we don't understand the exact mechanisms. The headaches are not necessarily the same as migraine but they are similar: severe, pulsating pain with nausea and vomiting, and made worse by movement.

Alcohol dilates blood vessels, affects blood sugar levels and increases the chemical prostaglandin – all of which cause headaches. It causes dehydration by affecting anti-diuretic hormones and it is broken down into acetaldehyde, which causes the skin flushing, nausea and vomiting associated with having a hangover.

Apart from avoiding alcohol, research doesn't show that there is anything that you can take to avoid getting a hangover. Treatment is simply rehydration and a couple of soluble painkillers. Coffee can sometimes help, but it is also dehydrating and can upset your stomach, so it may be best avoided. If you are going to drink alcohol, here are some tips to avoid headaches.

Tips for drinking alcohol and avoiding headaches

- Drink plenty of water and have something to eat.
- Drink alcohol slowly and in moderation.
- Avoid any drink that causes migraine quickly after a small amount – this may be a sensitivity rather than a hangover headache.
- Avoid top ups so that you can keep track of what you have had.
- Don't mix alcoholic drinks, which increases sensitivity in headache-prone people, regardless of amount.
- Beware of sparkling alcoholic drinks or even non-alcoholic mixers, which can speed up alcohol absorption.
- Avoid the risk associated with alcohol if you know that you are already vulnerable to a migraine attack because you are tired, have missed a meal or are stressed or excited.

Limit caffeine intake

Caffeine is a stimulant drug in coffee, tea, soft drinks and chocolate, which affects our brain by making us feel less tired and more alert. The relationship between caffeine and headache is complex. It can be added to paracetamol and aspirin tablets to enhance their painkiller effect. However, withdrawal from caffeine can cause severe headaches. For some people, caffeine intake is an additional risk factor for developing daily headaches.

Consider whether your caffeine intake could be contributing to your headaches. If you have more than 200 milligrams (mg) of caffeine daily and then stop or cut down, you can develop a caffeine withdrawal headache. Exact amounts of dietary caffeine are tricky to calculate. A cup of tea or can of soft drink may contain at least 40 mg, and a cup of coffee at least double that. It is more if the coffee is strong or you have a big mug! Add on 30 mg per chocolate bar and 30–65 mg *per tablet* of some of the combined painkillers, and you can see how easy it is for amounts to add up.

Research suggests that changes in brain blood flow account for caffeine withdrawal headaches. Anyone can have them – even people who don't normally have headaches. If you are very sensitive, then the difference in one cup of coffee a day is enough. If you drink fewer caffeinated drinks at the weekend than at work, weekend headaches may be due to caffeine withdrawal. They can be accompanied by restlessness, irritability and decreased alertness.

Tips for avoiding caffeine-related headache

- Minimize caffeine in your diet if you can.
- Choose decaffeinated options (only 5 mg per cup of coffee).
- Aim to keep low, stable levels of caffeine, even at weekends.
- Avoid caffeine in painkillers. Combination drugs with aspirin and paracetamol can lead to medication over-use more quickly.
- If you decide to cut down on your caffeine intake, do it very slowly over several weeks.

Dietary supplements

We have little evidence from clinical studies about what works and what is safe to use short or long term. Supplements have side effects, may interfere with other medications and should be discussed with your doctor.

Vitamin B₂ riboflavin

Some of the B-group vitamins have been postulated to be helpful in headaches and migraine. We have the best evidence for vitamin B_2 (riboflavin). This water-soluble vitamin is involved in releasing energy from the body's cells. Small research trials suggest high doses of 400 mg daily (this is at least 20 times the recommended daily intake) can be effective in preventing migraine. The dose should not be taken as part of a multivitamin preparation to avoid overdosing on other vitamins. Apart from bright yellow urine, side effects in the trials were minimal.

Magnesium

Magnesium has many functions in the body, including glucose metabolism, and it is one of the essential minerals. Research has shown some benefit for magnesium supplements in preventing migraine, particularly for women who also have premenstrual syndrome. The dosages range from 300 to 600 mg daily and ideally should be taken for a six-month course. Diarrhoea can be a side effect.

Coenzyme Q₁₀

Coenzyme Q_{10} occurs naturally in the body and speeds up the processes by which cells produce energy. Evidence from a small-scale study suggested that it could reduce the frequency of migraine attacks by up to half in some people. There were some side effects such as nausea, rashes and fatigue, but it was generally well tolerated. We need much more research but, if it is taken in single doses of up to 150–300 mg per day over several months, there may be some benefit. It can interfere with other medications such as warfarin and insulin.

5-Hydroxytryptophan

5-Hydroxytryptophan (5-HTP) is an amino acid in the body that is used to make the chemical messenger serotonin. This may be implicated in migraine. There is no robust evidence from clinical studies for benefit from 5-HTP supplements. They should not be taken if you use triptans to treat migraine because of a risk of serotonin toxicity (serotonin syndrome). It may be possible to boost your serotonin levels naturally in your diet. Carbohydrate-rich meals can increase serotonin, and some foods such as turkey are high in tryptophan, which is converted into serotonin.

Melatonin

Melatonin is a hormone released from the pineal gland in the brain, which regulates our sleep cycle. We need more research to establish whether it is safe and effective in preventing migraine and cluster headache. It should not be used for headaches outside clinical trials. We have little information on side effects, and it could adversely stimulate the immune system.

Herbal supplements

Herbal treatments have been used for centuries and are the origins of some of our conventional drugs today. Some people find them helpful for headaches but they should not be regarded as safe just because they are 'natural'. Herbal medicines can be highly toxic and interact with other medicines. The Medicines Health and Regulatory Authority in the UK increasingly register traditional herbs, but unlike conventional medicines there is no requirement to demonstrate that they work.

If you take a herbal approach to coping with headache, ideally consult a qualified herbalist for professional advice. (See Useful addresses at the end of this book.)

If you are currently using herbal supplements or considering them, here are some tips.

Tips on selecting and using herbal supplements

- Obtain as much information as you can.
- Purchase from a reputable source.
- Read labels so that you know what doses to take.
- Follow instructions carefully.
- Seek advice from your doctor, pharmacist or herbalist.
- Avoid taking several herbal medicines at the same time unless you are advised to do so.
- Use the lowest possible dose that works for you.
- Use herbal treatment for headache prevention for an agreed time and keep a diary to see if there is an improvement.
- Avoid long-term use because we do not have safety data.

Treatment with herbs can be by tablet, infusions, inhalations, warm compresses, massage oils and baths. Peppermint and lavender are commonly used for relief of headaches and migraine. Ginger, which is a spice, may help with associated nausea. It can be taken as tea, in biscuits or crystallized. The following herbal treatments have been used for migraine prevention.

Feverfew

Feverfew (*Tanecetum parthenium*) is part of the daisy family. Feverfew has been shown in some small trials to be better than placebo (dummy treatments) for reducing the number of migraine attacks. Other trials have not demonstrated an effect and larger studies are needed. We don't know exactly how it works, but it affects relaxation and contraction of blood vessels and stops release of serotonin from platelets, which could interfere with migraine mechanisms. The dose of tablets is 200–250 mg daily. It can also be taken as three or four fresh leaves daily, and the bitter taste can be disguised by eating it in a sandwich.

Let your doctor know if you want to use feverfew. You should not use it if you are pregnant, breastfeeding or taking aspirin or warfarin because of its blood thinning effects. Side effects include digestive upsets and mouth ulcers. You should try feverfew for three months because it can take over a month to start working. Long-term use cannot be recommended because we do not have any safety data.

Butterbur

Butterbur petasin (*Petasites hybridus*) is a native European perennial shrub. We have some evidence from small clinical trials that butterbur can help to prevent migraine attacks. The active ingredients extracted from the root are called petasin and isopetasin. They are believed to act as anti-inflammatories and have effects on blood vessels.

Butterbur capsules 25 mg can be taken twice daily. The supplements must be purchased from a reputable source to ensure removal of naturally occurring toxic components, which may cause liver damage and cancer. Butterbur appears to be well tolerated, with the main potential side effects being gastrointestinal such as nausea, vomiting, stomach pain and diarrhoea.

St John's wort

St John's wort (*Hypericum perforatum*) is a perennial herb. Used to treat mild to moderate depression, it affects serotonin levels. There is some clinical trial evidence for improving depression, but not specifically migraine. The trial doses ranged between 300 and 1050 mg daily. St John's wort interacts with a number of medications, including the triptans (anti-migraine), anti-depressants, anti-epileptics, contraceptives, asthma drugs, heart drugs and blood thinning drugs. You should not take St John's wort without discussing it with your doctor first. It is not recommended during pregnancy.

19

Non-drug strategies

Non-drug strategies are attractive because not every one wants to use medications for headaches. Drugs don't always work, they have side effects and they can be over-used. It is also important not to think only of a conventional drug-orientated approach. You should consider how your whole body and mind work together to optimize your health and influence your headaches.

Sadly, various non-drug devices on the market promise cures and invariably disappoint. Try them and hope that you are not wasting your money. In contrast, simple heat pads, ice packs and cooling strips can be effective. There are also physical and psychological strategies, which may be beneficial. Some are termed complementary therapies, which is a useful way to think of them – complementing medical treatments. If you can combine and integrate approaches, this may give you a greater chance of success than either on their own.

We do not have any definitive scientific proof that any of the following approaches work for headaches, despite considerable research in some areas. We cannot state that any one strategy is better than another – it is a matter of trying and finding something that works for you.

Physical strategies

Physical strategies can be effective in chronic tension-type headache, migraine and headaches that occur following trauma such as whiplash injury. The brain stem at the top of the neck joins the brain with the spinal cord, and the nerves here link to the muscles and joints of the neck. It is possible that treatment of the neck and spine influences not just mechanical function but also nervous system function, which could influence headaches and migraine.

Specific differences between physiotherapy, chiropractic and osteopathy are debatable, and techniques overlap. The practitioner should always provide a thorough initial assessment and advice on your treatment plan.

Physiotherapy

Manual therapy by a physiotherapist can alleviate problems associated with the neck and spine. Treatments include massage, mobilization, manipulation and correction of posture. Improvement of your physical well being can improve tension-type headaches and migraine. Some physiotherapists additionally offer acupuncture, lifestyle and stress management. This profession is allied to medicine, and physiotherapists in the UK are registered by the Chartered Society of Physiotherapy. (See Useful addresses at the end of this book.)

Osteopathy and chiropractic

These disciplines, like physiotherapy, are manual therapies that use various techniques such as manipulation of the bones and muscles. This manipulation ranges from gentle massage to short sharp thrusts to realign the spine and neck. The approaches are holistic, with the premise that good health is promoted when problems with the structure of the body are minimized. This can ensure good function of the whole body, including blood vessels and nerves.

Clinical trial evidence has not been conclusive. However, this approach may help migraine and especially tension-type headache, particularly if you have muscle spasm, pain, and tender points in your neck and shoulders that can trigger your headache. Osteopathy and chiropractic are the only two complementary therapies that are fully regulated, like medicine and physiotherapy. (See Useful addresses at the end of this book). Some practitioners specialize in cranial osteopathy, which concentrates on gentle manipulation of the skull. This is controversial with no scientific basis. If therapists are not called osteopaths, then they will not necessarily be members of the fully regulated healthcare profession.

Exercise

There have been few studies assessing the benefit of exercise on headache and migraine. They have been small and did not last very long, so we do not know whether any supposed benefits were maintained. We need larger scale and longer term research. Exercise is good for your general health because it improves blood pressure, obesity, heart disease risk factors and physical fitness, and it reduces risk of diabetes and depression. How exercise may help prevent migraine and tension-type headache is not known. It could be due to increases in endorphins (the body's natural painkillers) and improved blood flow in the body.

Some people with migraine avoid exercise because it can be a trigger for headache. However, if you are strict about a proper warm up, exercise within a comfortable level for your own fitness, drink plenty of fluids and maintain blood sugar levels before, during and after exercise, then headaches can often be avoided. Joining a gym and having personal training sessions may suit some people but this can be expensive. Bouts of exercise – even just brisk walking for ten minutes at a time, three times a day – all add up. If you can manage this five days a week then you can improve your general fitness. If you can incorporate this into your routine, it may be easier than going to the gym. It is best if you enjoy what you do, so that you can maintain it as part of your healthy lifestyle.

Alexander technique

This technique, formulated around 1900, focuses on your perception of your body's movement and posture through physical and psychological principles. Improvement of stiff and painful shoulders, neck or back, for example, may have a positive effect on your headache. It can be learnt from a teacher in a group or individual session and takes commitment to learn and perfect.

Yoga

Originating in India, this incorporates physical and mental techniques, which can promote relaxation, stress reduction and ease muscular tension. There are many types and they may help prevent some headache triggers. Breathing exercises can be useful during an attack of migraine. You need to be taught by a qualified teacher and take time to learn at your own pace.

Pilates

This uses controlled breathing to align the spine and strengthen muscles. The movements aim to be controlled and precise. Gentle exercises, which can be performed at your own pace within a class, can promote a feeling of improved health and well being.

Massage, aromatherapy and reflexology

Massage may reduce anxiety and muscle tension and promote better sleep, which could help with migraine and headache. Oils rubbed onto the skin during aromatherapy massage or inhaled must be used with care because strong smells can trigger migraine. Essential oils should be diluted in a 'carrier oil'. We have no idea of the safety and toxicity of strong oils used over long periods of time. So short-term use of three to six months is sensible, and they should not be used if you are pregnant. Peppermint, lavender and eucalyptus are often suggested for treatment of headaches and migraine. Try one a time to see whether any are effective for you. In reflexology the foot is massaged to promote improvement in health. Although there is no scientific evidence for this therapy for any conditions, it can be very relaxing and people with headaches may respond positively.

Transcutaneous electrical nerve stimulation

Transcutaneous electrical nerve stimulation (TENS) devices are used to control pain. They generate a small electric current, which can override pain message transmission to the brain. Studies have not shown significant benefits for people with headaches and migraine, but TENS may be useful alongside other therapies, particularly if you have back or neck problems.

Dental treatment

If you clench your jaw, grind your teeth (bruxism), or have an over-bite or a misalignment of your teeth (malocclusion), then these can cause jaw pain and muscular tension. Chewing gum can make problems worse. There is no robust evidence to suggest that splints or mouth guards can help with tension-type headache and migraine. However, it is worth asking your dentist for their opinion, because some people find headaches improve if these problems are corrected.

Psychological strategies

This approach focuses on positive thinking, reducing stress and anxiety, promoting relaxation and coping better with headache pain. These techniques and therapies are useful if you have depression and anxiety in addition to headaches, but they can benefit everyone.

Cognitive behavioural therapy

Cognitive behavioural therapy (CBT) is a psychotherapy approach that helps you to think about relationships between stress, headaches and coping. Learning how to change unhelpful thoughts and behaviours with CBT may enable you to control how you respond to stress, even if you cannot change the circumstances. This can be helpful to stop migraine triggers, change your lifestyle and reduce anxiety. It focuses on the present and challenges feelings of depression, helplessness and a 'just keep taking the tablets' approach. You can deal with your headaches in a more positive way and take more control. For example, rather than staying in worrying about developing a headache, you can learn to think, 'I might get a headache, but it isn't going to stop me from going out. If I get one I'll deal with it.'

There are some online programmes that you can work through, but ideally you should work with a qualified psychologist. Sessions last about an hour and around ten may be required. You can be referred by your doctor, or find a therapist yourself. It can be quite challenging but worthwhile.

Relaxation

Any relaxation technique that can help reduce stress and anxiety may be beneficial in preventing migraine and tension-type headache by raising your threshold for developing them. Relaxation exercises can also distract you from a headache that has begun.

We don't know the exact mechanism underlying the relation between stress and headache. Stress rarely causes headaches but there is an association, and people often notice that migraine occurs with relaxation after a stressful event. Although we don't have much evidence, relaxation could mean lower levels of tension, which could make us more resistant to the stress response. That means that by being able to relax more, you reduce stress chemicals circulating in your body.

You can learn relaxation techniques such as deep breathing, meditation or visualization from CDs and DVDs. They can also be learned as part of disciplines such as yoga. Other relaxation techniques such as biofeedback and self-hypnosis are best learned from a therapist. All of these take commitment to learn and time to practice. If you can learn to relax more and balance some of the highs and lows of stressful everyday living, this could help with your headaches.

Biofeedback

Biofeedback training teaches you to control unconscious processes in your body that you are not normally aware of. These include hand temperature, heart rate and muscular tension. Techniques are taught by psychologists during several sessions using a computer to monitor your temperature, muscle activity or brain waves, depending on which biofeedback you are learning. With practice you can use the techniques at any time. There is some research evidence that the relaxation involved reduces stress, and the calming effect can help some people to control their headaches. Contact the headache organizations for details of where biofeedback is taught. (See Useful addresses at the end of this book.)

Hypnotherapy

Hypnotherapy or hypnosis achieves a deep relaxation state in which you subconsciously learn to change the way you feel about pain. Your body learns different ways of responding. Under the guidance of a qualified therapist you can learn self-hypnosis techniques. You may be able to reduce the frequency of headaches by raising your threshold or possibly stop headaches worsening when they start. We have no research evidence to prove that this therapy is effective, but some people may find it helpful.

Other complementary therapies

There are many complementary therapies available. The main ones that have been subjected to clinical study for headache are acupuncture and homeopathy.

Acupuncture

This is the traditional ancient Chinese practice of inserting fine needles into certain points of your body. The needles tap into energy channels with the aim of promoting healing and restoring balance. Western medical acupuncture uses needles at specific points to influence pain mechanisms. The body's natural painkillers (endorphins) may be released during the needling process. The benefits of acupuncture in headache prevention have been studied, but the results are debated and more trials are needed. Acupuncture may be helpful if you have a course with a qualified practitioner. (See Useful addresses at the end of this book). You may need to repeat treatments to maintain any improvement. You can try acupressure yourself by pressing with your fingers on tender points such as your temple and neck.

Homeopathy

This method of therapy is based on principles of using substances in very dilute preparations to treat 'like with like'. A qualified homeopathic practitioner determines what is required based on individual needs. Clinical trials have shown very mixed results in headache. It may help some people and can be used alongside conventional medicine. A qualified practitioner is always preferable to trying over-the-counter remedies.

Tips for using non-drug strategies

- Do some investigating first. Read about likely effects of treatments so that you can ask informed questions.
- Be wary of any approach offering a cure. Some are based on testimonials from a few people gained by offering cut price treatments and are worthless.
- Consider carefully before parting with money. Many treatments are not available on the National Health Service because they have not been shown to work and can prove expensive over time.
- Choose your therapist with care. Ensure that they are registered or accredited if appropriate. (See Useful addresses at the end of this book.)
- Getting effective therapy involves working with your therapist. Do not commit before you are ready to.
- Tell your therapist about your medical history including medications that you are taking. A holistic approach can help with your general health, not just with your headache.
- Have realistic expectations, because you cannot expect never to have a headache again. However, if your headache or general health improves, then that is an important benefit. Sometimes just taking time out from a busy life can be helpful.
- Keep a diary record of your headache to assess effectiveness.
- Ask your therapist whether headaches may get worse before they improve. This can happen and it is best to be prepared.
- Ask your therapist how long a course of treatment is likely to take. As with all prevention strategies, give it long enough to work.
- Don't try too many things at once – otherwise you can't be sure what works and what doesn't.
- Don't change medications without discussing with your general practitioner and let them know what other strategies you are trying.

20

Help from your doctor

A supportive doctor is an ally, yet only around three per cent of us see our doctor specifically about headaches each year. Headaches are under-diagnosed and under-treated, and coping with headaches continues to be a burden that many people bear alone. If you can combine self-help strategies with the ongoing support of your doctor, you may gain better control over your headaches.

Do you need to go to the doctor?

If you have any of the signs or symptoms covered in Chapter 1, see your doctor to check the diagnosis. Aside from these features, you do not necessarily need to see a doctor unless you are concerned or need more help. Whether you choose to seek medical help is a personal decision. The doctor who gives you the support you need may not be the first one you meet.

Having a medical opinion helps you to understand your headaches. Information from a book or the internet cannot replace a personal consultation, and it is always reassuring when serious causes for a headache are ruled out. This can be therapy in its own right – it doesn't have to be about taking medications.

Your doctor can also help you with any other medical conditions that you might not connect with your headaches but could be making them worse. (See Chapter 17.)

Realistic expectations

It is important not to expect a cure for headache, because this is unlikely and will always be disappointing. Similarly, don't expect dramatic improvement after a single visit. It is more likely that several visits, months apart, will be required to optimize treatment. The reality is that headache management can be trial and error until you find something that suits you. Even then, don't be alarmed if your needs change and strategies require reassessment in the future.

You should expect your doctor to work with you and be able to discuss your expectations and concerns in an open way. These are different for different people. It might be about improving pain control, reducing frequency, stopping medication over-use or just reassurance that nothing is wrong. Your doctor should be sympathetic and explain your headache and possible management options in a way that you can understand. Together, you can make a decision about what is best for you.

Information the doctor will need

Apart from questions about other illnesses and general lifestyle, your doctor needs to find out about your headaches. There are different styles of consultation. Some doctors let you describe your headaches without interruption, but others ask you structured questions about each kind of headache you have. Obtaining this information is important for diagnosis and deciding whether further examination and investigation are necessary.

Before you see a doctor it is helpful to have an idea of the questions you may be asked or the information that you would like to give. Here are some ideas based on recommendations by the British Association for the Study of Headache. Think about them for each type of headache, if you have more than one.

Time questions

- When did your headache start? How long does it last? How often do you get it?
- Have you had a headache like this before?

Character of headache questions

- How severe is the pain? What is it like? Where is it? Does it spread anywhere else?
- Do you have any other symptoms before, during or after the pain?

Cause of headache questions

- Have you noticed any triggering factors, any aggravating factors or any relieving factors?
- Does anyone in your family have a similar headache or have they done so in the past?

Your response to the headache questions

- What do you prefer to do during the headache?
- Are your usual activities at home/work/school limited or prevented by the headache?
- Are you using medications now for your headache? Do they work? What have you tried in the past and did they work?
- What other treatments or strategies have you tried and did they help?

General health question

- Are you completely well between headaches or are there any persisting symptoms?

Other questions

- Why are you seeking help now?
- Has your headache become worse or changed?
- Do you have any concerns about the headache and its cause?
- Is there any other information that you would like to give about your headache?

Examination by the doctor

The first time you see a doctor or specialist about your headache, they will usually examine you. This is straightforward and undressing isn't normally necessary. People often wonder why doctors don't do more detailed examinations for headache. This is because they obtain most of the information required for diagnosis from your headache history. The examination allows your doctor to confirm the diagnosis, and is typically normal if you have a primary headache.

Your doctor will usually take your blood pressure. Although raised blood pressure isn't a usual cause of headaches, it may influence the choice of treatment. The doctor will examine your eyes using a torch-like device (ophthalmoscope). Increased pressure in the brain can cause headache and swelling, which may be seen in the back of the eye. The doctor will also assess your field of vision and eye movements to check that specific nerves in the brain are functioning correctly. Additionally, the doctor may feel your head and neck muscles to check for tenderness, which is often present in tension-type headache and migraine. They will also listen to your chest and neck using a stethoscope. This assesses your heart and blood flow to your brain.

The doctor may do various simple tests to check your co-ordination and reflexes, for example walking on your heels and toes and touching your nose with your finger. These are quick and easy but effective ways of checking different nerve pathways from your brain throughout your body – rather like a physical brain scan. These tests do not reveal any problem in most people with headaches. If your doctor is uncertain about the diagnosis then they may do further investigations.

Investigations and tests

There are no blood tests, radiographs (x-ray scans) or brain scans that show that you have migraine, tension-type headache or cluster headache. The results are normal. This surprises many people, who think a brain scan is essential – probably because their headache makes them feel so ill. Although a brain scan can be reassuring to both you and your doctor, it doesn't necessarily help him or her to diagnose the headache.

If there is doubt about the diagnosis and other causes of headaches must be ruled out, or you have a rare type of headache such as cluster headache, then your doctor may do further tests. If you have had a head injury, your doctor may order a skull x-ray scan. Blood tests may be useful if your doctor suspects headache due to infection or other diseases.

There are two main types of brain scans. CT (computed tomography) scans can detect bleeding, tumours and blood vessel abnormalities. MRI (magnetic resonance imaging) scans show all the blood vessels and brain tissue extremely clearly and may be used to detect strokes and very small tumours. If your doctor sends you for a scan, they are not necessarily sure that you have a serious cause for your headache, but they want to eliminate the possibility and confirm the diagnosis.

Headache specialist referral

Specialist referral for headaches is either to a neurologist (a doctor who specializes in disorders of the nervous system) or to a headache clinic. These are usually run by neurologists, general practitioners with a special interest in headache or specialist nurse practitioners. There are headache clinics in the UK that can provide advice on all aspects of headache management. (See Useful addresses at the end of this book.)

Your doctor may refer you if your headache diagnosis is not clear or if your response to standard treatment is not as expected. If you have cluster headache, then specialist referral is recommended to ensure that your treatment is optimized urgently. Early referral of trouble-some headaches to a specialist is always best. Because it is possible to have more than one kind of headache, sometimes a specialist opinion is helpful. It is not always straightforward to determine whether you have one type or multiple types of headache – even for specialists. The specialist will liaise with your doctor with their recommendations.

Other referrals

Because headaches are influenced by many factors, your doctor may refer you to other healthcare professionals, including physiotherapists, psychologists or pain specialists. Pain clinics can help you to combine various techniques. This doesn't mean just medications, but includes CBT (cognitive behavioural therapy) together with TENS (transcuta-neous electrical nerve stimulation). Combinations of strategies may be beneficial if you have had severe headaches for a long time or if you have other pain conditions as well.

'Off-label' prescriptions

If you need medication for headaches, your doctor can prescribe many more options than those available over-the-counter. These include medications that are specifically licensed to treat headaches and also those that are not but have still been found to be very effective. These include medications commonly used for blood pressure, depression, heart problems and epilepsy. If your doctor or specialist prescribes these medications 'off-label', then this will be explained to you and noted in your record. Their use is widely accepted in tackling headache and includes some of our useful treatments, such as amitryptyline in migraine and tension-type headache and verapamil and oxygen in cluster headache.

Tips for getting medical help

- Although many people don't go to their doctor with headaches (or have given up), if you are unable to cope on your own seek help.
- If your doctor is not sympathetic or providing support (despite your realistic expectations), then see a different one or go to a specialist clinic. Not all clinics require a doctor's referral. At the City of London Migraine Clinic you can refer yourself for an appointment. (See Useful addresses at the end of this book.) Don't give up!
- If you don't understand, ask again. You will cope much better with new strategies if you understand what they are for and what to expect. Doctors are usually happy to write things down, give you a copy of letters or provide an information leaflet.
- Make some notes yourself. If your doctor is recommending combining or changing treatments, the regimen can be complex. You don't want to be wondering what you should be doing with your tablets in the middle of a migraine attack!
- Take your partner or a friend to the consultation. What one of you forgets, the other might remember. Involving your partner helps them to understand, so that they can support you.
- Prepare for the appointment by thinking about questions you might be asked.
- Take a headache diary to the appointment or keep a diary if requested.
- Be proactive in managing your headache. You may need to be prepared to make changes to your lifestyle and to try new treatments and give them a fair trial.
- Tell your doctor if you are working with other healthcare professionals and therapists or using other treatments. Even some over-the-counter preparations can interact with prescription medicines.
- Let your doctor know whether treatments are effective. If, after a proper trial, something doesn't work for you, then your doctor may suggest something else, rethink the diagnosis or refer you to a specialist clinic.

Further reading

UK guidelines for management of headaches

British Association for the Study of Headache (BASH)
Steiner TJ, MacGregor EA, Davies PTG. *Guidelines for all Healthcare Professionals in the Diagnosis and Management of Migraine, Tension-type, Cluster and Medication Overuse Headache.* BASH, 2007. (Available from www.bash.org)

Scottish Intercollegiate Guidelines Network (SIGN)
SIGN. *Diagnosis and management of headache in adults. A national clinical guideline.* SIGN, 2008. (Available from www.sign.ac.uk)

Journal articles

Cohen A, Matharu M, Goadsby PJ. 'Trigeminal autonomic cephalalgias: current and future treatments.' *Headache* 2007, 47:969–980. (Article on cluster headache.)

Diener H-C, Limmroth V. 'Medication-overuse headache: a worldwide problem.' *Lancet Neurol* 2004, 3:475–483.

Evans EW, Lorber KC. 'Use of 5-HT1 agonists in pregnancy.' *Ann Pharmacother* 2008, 42:543–549. (Article on triptan use in pregnancy.)

Goadsby PJG. 'Recent advances in the diagnosis and management of migraine.' *BMJ* 2006, 332:25–29.

Katsarava Z, Jensen R. 'Medication-overuse headache: where are we now?' *Curr Opin Neurol* 2007, 20:326–330.

Lipton RB, Dodick D, Sadovsky R, *et al.* 'A self-administered screener for migraine in primary care: the ID Migraine™ validation study.' *Neurology* 2003, 61:375–382.

Loder E, Rizzoli P. 'Tension-type headache.' *BMJ* 2008, 336:88–92.

MacGregor EA, Frith A, Ellis J, *et al.* 'Predicting menstrual migraine with a home-use fertility monitor.' *Neurology* 2005, 64:561–563.

MacGregor EA. 'Migraine in pregnancy and lactation: a clinical review.' *J Fam Plann Reprod Health Care* 2007, 33:83–93.

Steiner TJ, Fontebasso M. 'Headache.' *BMJ* 2002, 325:881–886.

Steiner TJ, Scher AI, Stewart WF, *et al.* 'The prevalence and disability burden of adult migraine in England and their relationships to age, gender and ethnicity.' *Cephalalgia* 2003, 23:519–527.

Stovner LJ, Hagen K, Jensen R, *et al.* 'The global burden of headache: a documentation of headache prevalence and disability worldwide.' *Cephalalgia* 2007, 27:193–210.

Books

Dryden W. *Letting Go of Anxiety and Depression*. Sheldon Press, London, 2003.

Hutchinson S, Peterlin BL (eds). *Menstrual Migraine*. Oxford American Pain Library, Oxford, 2008.

Kernick D, Goadsby PJ (eds). *Headache: a Practical Manual*. Oxford University Press, Oxford, 2009.

MacGregor A. *Understanding Menopause and HRT*. Family Doctor Publications, Poole, 2007.

MacGregor A, Frith A (eds). *ABC of Headache*. Wiley-Blackwell BMJ Books, Chichester, 2009.

Useful addresses

Specialist headache clinic

The City of London Migraine Clinic
22 Charterhouse Square
London EC1M 6DX
Tel: 020 7251 3322
Website: www.migraineclinic.org.uk

An independent medical charity providing help for migraine, cluster headache and other types of headache by appointment with specialist doctors. There are opportunities to take part in research. Diaries and factsheets can be downloaded from the website. Self-referral is accepted by telephone or via the website, or you can be referred by your doctor. A donation per clinic visit is suggested from UK residents, and non-UK residents can be seen privately – contact the clinic for details.

Information and helpline support for headaches

The following organizations provide excellent information on their websites and in their newsletters. They run helplines and, if you need medical advice, they can supply details of headache clinics near where you live. They support and fund research and raise awareness of migraine and headaches.

Migraine Action
Fourth Floor
27 East Street
Leicester LE1 6NB
Tel: 0116 275 8317 (also helpline)
Website: www.migraine.org.uk

Migraine Association of Ireland
Unit 14, Block 5
Port Tunnel Business Park
Clonshaugh
Dublin 17
Tel: 00 353 1 8941280 or 01 8941281
Callsave helpline: 1850 200 378 (ROI); 0844 826 9323 (NI)
Website: www.migraine.ie

The Migraine Trust
55–56 Russell Square
London WC1B 4HP
Tel: 020 7436 1336
Information and Enquiries: 020 7462 6601
Website: www.migrainetrust.org

OUCH (UK)
Organization for the Understanding of Cluster Headache
74 Abbotsbury Road
Broadstone
Dorset BH18 9DD
Helpline: 01646 651 979
Website: www.ouchuk.org

Headache organization websites

The following organizations are dedicated to promoting a better understanding of headache, and their websites provide useful information and links for the public and healthcare professionals. Membership of some is open only to professionals working in the headache field.

American Headache Society
www.americanheadachesociety.org

British Association for the Study of Headache (BASH)
www.bash.org.uk

European Headache Federation
www.ehf-org.org

International Headache Society (IHS)
www.i-h-s.org

Lifting the Burden: The Global Campaign to Reduce the Burden of Headache Worldwide
www.l-t-b.org

Migraine Action Plan
www.migraineactionplan.co.uk

Migraine in Primary Care Advisors (MIPCA)
www.mipca.org.uk

World Headache Alliance
www.w-h-a.org

Health addresses and websites

Menopause Matters
www.menopausematters.co.uk

An independent, clinician-led website providing information about the
menopause and all the treatment options.

Mental Health Foundation
London Office, 9th Floor
Sea Containers House
20 Upper Ground
London SE1 9QB
Tel: 020 7803 1101
Website: www.mentalhealth.org.uk

National Association for Premenstrual Syndrome
41 Old Road
East Peckham
Kent TN12 5AP
Tel: 0870 777 2178
Website: www.pms.org.uk

New You
Website: www.new-you.tv

An online TV resource providing information and videos on current
health issues, including migraine and headaches.

NHS Direct
Tel: 0845 4647
Website: www.nhsdirect.nhs.uk

The 24-hour telephone helpline for nurse advice and health information
if you are unwell. Since November 2008, NHS Direct has been linked to
NHS Choices (<www.nhs.uk>) to provide all NHS information under one
website.

Patient UK
Website: www.patient.co.uk

An information resource on a wide range of health topics, including
migraine and headaches.

Smokefree
Tel: 0800 022 4 332 (7 a.m. to 11 p.m. every day of the year)
Website: http://smokefree.nhs.uk

NHS free smoking helpline.

Therapy practitioner information

The following organizations provide information on various therapies and disciplines and have lists of registered practitioners.

The Aromatherapy Council
PO Box 6522
Desborough
Northants NN14 2YX
Tel: 0870 774 3477
Website: www.aromatherapycouncil.org.uk

Body Control Pilates
35 Little Russell Street
London WC1A 2HH
Tel: 020 7636 8900
Website: www.bodycontrol.co.uk

British Acupuncture Council
63 Jeddo Road
London W12 9HQ
Tel: 020 8735 0400
Website: www.acupuncture.org.uk

British Association for Behavioural and Cognitive Psychotherapies (BABCP)
Victoria Buildings
9–13 Silver Street
Bury BL9 0EU
Tel: 0161 797 4484
Website: www.babcp.com

British Association for Applied Nutrition and Nutritional Therapy
27 Old Gloucester Street
London WC1N 3XX
Tel: 0870 606 1284
Website: www.bant.org.uk

British Association for Counselling and Psychotherapy
BACP House
15 St John's Business Park
Kutterworth
Leics LE17 4HB
Tel: 01455 883 316
Website: www.bacp.co.uk

British Chiropractic Association
59 Castle Street
Reading
Berkshire RG1 7SN
Tel: 0118 950 5950
Website: www.chiropractic-uk.co.uk

British Complementary Medicine Association (BCMA)
PO Box 5122
Bournemouth BH8 0WG
Tel: 0845 345 5977
Website: www.bcma.co.uk

British Homeopathic Association
Hahnemann House
29 Park Street West
Luton LU1 3BE
Tel: 01582 408675
Website: www.trusthomeopathy.org

British Hypnotherapy Association
30 Cotsford Avenue
New Malden
Surrey KT3 5EU
Tel: 020 8579 5533/020 8942 3988
Website: www.british-hypnotherapy-association.org

British Medical Acupuncture Society
BMAS House
3 Winnington Court
Northwich
Cheshire CW8 1AQ
Tel: 01606 786782
Website: www.medical-acupuncture.co.uk

British Psychological Society (BPS)
St Andrew's House
48 Princess Road East
Leicester LE1 7DR
Tel: 0116 254 9568
Website: www.bps.org.uk

British Reflexology Association
Monks Orchard
Whitbourne
Worcester WR6 5RB
Tel: 01886 821207
Website: www.britreflex.org.uk

British Society of Clinical and Academic Hypnosis
National Office Secretary
28 Dale Park Gardens
Cookridge
Leeds LS16 7PT
Tel: 0844 884 3116
Website: www.bscah.com

British Wheel of Yoga
BWY Central Office
25 Jermyn Street
Sleaford
Lincolnshire NG34 7RU
Tel: 01529 306851
Website: www.bwy.org.uk

Chartered Society of Physiotherapy
14 Bedford Row
London WC1R 4ED
Tel: 020 7306 6666
Website: www.csp.org.uk

General Osteopathic Council
176 Tower Bridge Road
London SE1 3LU
Tel: 020 7357 6655
Website: www.osteopathy.org.uk

Institute for Complementary Medicine and Natural Medicine
Can-Mezzanine
32–36 Loman Street
London SE1 0EH
Tel: 020 7922 7980
Website: www.i-c-m.org.uk

National Institute of Medical Herbalists
Elm House
54 Mary Arches Street
Exeter EX4 3BA
Tel: 01392 426022
Website: www.nimh.org.uk

Relaxation for Living Institute
1 Great Chapel Street
London W1F 8FA
Tel: 020 9671 1724
Website: www.rfli.co.uk

Society of Teachers of the Alexander Technique
First Floor, Linton House
39–51 Highgate Road
London NW5 1RS
Tel: 0845 230 7828 (10 a.m. to 5 p.m., Monday to Friday)
Website: www.stat.org.uk

United Kingdom Council of Psychotherapy
Second Floor, Edward House
2 Wakley Street
London EC1V 7LT
Tel: 020 7014 9955
Website: www.ukcp.org.uk

Index